Clinical Management of Neuroendocrine Tumors of the Lung

Editor

PIER LUIGI FILOSSO

THORACIC
SURGERY CLINICS

www.thoracic.theclinics.com

Consulting Editor
M. BLAIR MARSHALL

August 2014 • Volume 24 • Number 3

ELSEVIER

1600 John F. Kennedy Boulevard • Suite 1800 • Philadelphia, Pennsylvania, 19103-2899

http://www.thoracic.theclinics.com

THORACIC SURGERY CLINICS Volume 24, Number 3
August 2014 ISSN 1547-4127, ISBN-13: 978-0-323-32026-9

Editor: John Vassallo (j.vassallo@elsevier.com)
Developmental Editor: Stephanie Carter

Thoracic Surgery Clinics (ISSN 1547-4127) is published quarterly by Elsevier Inc., 360 Park Avenue South, New York, NY 10010-1710. Months of publication are February, May, August, and November. Business and editorial offices: 1600 John F. Kennedy Boulevard, Suite 1800, Philadelphia, PA 19103-2899. Periodicals postage paid at New York, NY, and additional mailing offices. Subscription prices are $350.00 per year (US individuals), $453.00 per year (US institutions), $165.00 per year (US Students), $435.00 per year (Canadian individuals), $585.00 per year (Canadian institutions), $225.00 per year (Canadian and foreign students), $465.00 per year (foreign individuals), and $585.00 per year (foreign institutions). Foreign air speed delivery is included in all Clinics' subscription prices. All prices are subject to change without notice. **POSTMASTER:** Send address changes to Thoracic Surgery Clinics, Elsevier Health Sciences Division, Subscription Customer Service, 3251 Riverport Lane, Maryland Heights, MO 63043. **Customer Service (orders, claims, online, change of address): Telephone: 1-800-654-2452 (U.S. and Canada); 314-447-8871 (outside U.S. and Canada). Fax: 314-447-8029. E-mail: journalscustomerservice-usa@elsevier.com (for print support); journalsonlinesupport-usa@elsevier.com (for online support).**

Reprints. For copies of 100 or more, of articles in this publication, please contact Commercial Rights Department, Elsevier Inc., 360 Park Avenue South, New York, NY 10010-1710. Tel: 212-633-3874; Fax: 212-633-3820; E-mail: reprints@elsevier.com.

Thoracic Surgery Clinics is covered in *MEDLINE/PubMed (Index Medicus), EMBASE/Excerpta Medica, Science Citation Index Expanded (SciSearch®), Journal Citation Reports/Science Edition,* and *Current Contents®/Clinical Medicine.*

Contributors

CONSULTING EDITOR

M. BLAIR MARSHALL, MD
Associate Professor of Surgery, Georgetown
University School of Medicine; Chief, Division
of Thoracic Surgery, Department of Surgery,
Georgetown University Medical Center,
Washington, DC

EDITOR

PIER LUIGI FILOSSO, MD, FECTS, FCCP
Assistant Professor, Department of Thoracic
Surgery, University of Torino, San Giovanni
Battista Hospital, Torino, Italy

AUTHORS

MANUELA ALBERTELLI, MD, PhD
Endocrinology Unit, Department of Internal
Medicine and Medical Specialties, Center of
Excellence for Biomedical Research, IRCCS
AOU San Martino-IST, University of Genoa,
Genoa, Italy

MARCO ANILE, MD
Department of Thoracic Surgery, University of
Rome Sapienza, Rome, Italy

HISAO ASAMURA, MD
Division of Thoracic Surgery, National Cancer
Center Hospital, Chuo-ku, Tokyo, Japan

LISA BODEI, MD, PhD
Division of Nuclear Medicine, European
Institute of Oncology, Milan, Italy

ALESSANDRO BRUNELLI, MD
Department of Thoracic Surgery, St James's
University Hospital, Leeds, United Kingdom

ALFREDO CESARIO, MD
Deputy Scientific Director, Scientific Direction,
IRCCS-San Raffaele Pisana, Rome, Italy

MARTA CREMONESI, PhD
Division of Health Physics, European Institute
of Oncology, Milan, Italy

FRANK C. DETTERBECK, MD
Professor and Chief, Yale Thoracic Surgery,
Yale University, New Haven, Connecticut

DANIELE DISO, MD
Department of Thoracic Surgery, University
of Rome Sapienza, Rome, Italy

PIERO FEROLLA, MD, PhD
Multidisciplinary Group for Diagnosis and
Therapy of Neuroendocrine Tumors, ENETS
Center of Excellence, Umbria Regional
Cancer Network, Perugia, Italy

DIEGO FERONE, MD, PhD
Endocrinology Unit, Department of Internal
Medicine and Medical Specialties, Center of
Excellence for Biomedical Research, IRCCS
AOU San Martino-IST, University of Genoa,
Genoa, Italy

ANGELINA FILICE, MD
Department of Nuclear Medicine,
IRCCS-Arcispedale Santa Maria Nuova,
Reggio Emilia, Italy

PIER LUIGI FILOSSO, MD, FECTS, FCCP
Assistant Professor, Department of Thoracic
Surgery, University of Torino, San Giovanni
Battista Hospital, Torino, Italy

MARIANO GARCÍA-YUSTE, MD, PhD
Head of Thoracic Surgery, University Hospital
of Valladolid, Professor of Thoracic Surgery,
Valladolid University, Valladolid, Spain

CHIARA M. GRANA, MD
Division of Nuclear Medicine, European
Institute of Oncology, Milan, Italy

FRANCESCO GUERRERA, MD
Department of Thoracic Surgery, University
of Torino, Torino, Italy

MARK KIDD, PhD
Department of Surgery, Yale School of
Medicine, New Haven, Connecticut

PAOLO OLIVO LAUSI, MD
Department of Thoracic Surgery, University
of Torino, Torino, Italy

FILIPPO LOCOCO, MD
Unit of Thoracic Surgery, Department
of Nuclear Medicine, IRCCS-Arcispedale
Santa Maria Nuova, Reggio Emilia, Italy

JOSÉ MARÍA MATILLA, MD, PhD
Thoracic Surgeon, University Hospital of
Valladolid, Valladolid, Spain

**IRVIN M. MODLIN, MD, PhD, DSc, MA, FRCS
(Eng. & Ed), FCS (SA)**
Emeritus Professor, Department of Surgery,
Yale School of Medicine, New Haven,
Connecticut; Wren Laboratories; Clifton Life
Sciences, Branford, Connecticut

ALBERTO OLIARO, MD
Department of Thoracic Surgery, University
of Torino, Torino, Italy

MASSIMILIANO PACI, MD
Unit of Thoracic Surgery, Department of
Nuclear Medicine, IRCCS-Arcispedale Santa
Maria Nuova, Reggio Emilia, Italy

GIOVANNI PAGANELLI, MD
Division of Nuclear Medicine, European
Institute of Oncology, Milan; Radiometabolic
Unit, Department of Nuclear Medicine,
IRST-IRCCS, Meldola, Italy

MAJED REFAI, MD
Unit of Thoracic Surgery, Ospedali Riuniti,
Ancona, Italy

ERINO A. RENDINA, MD
Department of Thoracic Surgery, University
of Rome Sapienza, Rome, Italy

ENRICO RUFFINI, MD
Department of Thoracic Surgery, University
of Torino, Torino, Italy

HIROYUKI SAKURAI, MD
Division of Thoracic Surgery, National Cancer
Center Hospital, Chuo-ku, Tokyo, Japan

STEFANO SEVERI, MD
Radiometabolic Unit, Department of
Nuclear Medicine, IRST-IRCCS,
Meldola, Italy

GEORGIOS STAMATIS, MD
Professor of Surgery, Thoracic Surgery and
Endoscopy, Ruhrlandklinik, West German
Lung Center, University of Duisburg-Essen,
Essen, Germany

WILLIAM D. TRAVIS, MD
Attending Thoracic Pathologist,
Department of Pathology, Memorial
Sloan Kettering Cancer Center, New York,
New York

GIORGIO TREGLIA, MD
Department of Nuclear Medicine, Oncology
Institute of Southern Switzerland, Bellinzona,
Switzerland

FEDERICO VENUTA, MD
Department of Thoracic Surgery, University of
Rome Sapienza, Rome, Italy

ANNIBALE VERSARI, MD
Department of Nuclear Medicine,
IRCCS-Arcispedale Santa Maria Nuova,
Reggio Emilia, Italy

Contents

In the three-quarters of a century that have elapsed since the first description of a bronchial carcinoid, the field has progressed from serendipitous radiological or bronchoscopic diagnosis to computed tomography, magnetic resonance imaging, and somatostatin receptor imaging identification. Similarly, pathologic techniques have advanced from a naïve assessment of neoplasia to a delineation of several tumor subtypes and an understanding of the neuroendocrine basis of the disease process. A key unresolved question is the identification of the genetic and environmental activators that are responsible for the initiation of pulmonary neuroendocrine cell proliferation and neoplastic transformation.

Neuroendocrine (NE) tumors of the lung include a spectrum from low-grade typical carcinoid (TC) and intermediate-grade atypical carcinoid (AC) to high-grade large cell neuroendocrine carcinoma (LCNEC) and small cell lung carcinoma (SCLC). Although NE lung tumors are frequently discussed together, as in this article, carcinoids are very different from high-grade SCLC and LCNEC. SCLC and LCNEC are found in heavy-smoking, older patients, whereas smoking is not strongly associated with carcinoid tumors. On a molecular level, SCLC and LCNEC have extensive genetic abnormalities, but there are few in TC and slightly more in AC.

Neuroendocrine tumors of the lung encompass a wide spectrum. A carcinoid tumor is either a central smooth endobronchial tumor or a round, well-circumscribed, peripheral parenchymal lesion. Distinguishing typical carcinoid tumors from atypical carcinoid tumors is unreliable from a limited biopsy but can be based on age, presentation, and node enlargement. Large cell neuroendocrine cancer presents similarly to most non-small cell lung cancers. Small cell lung cancer has a characteristic presentation, with a rapid progression of symptoms, and a bulky central and/or mediastinal tumor. A diagnosis is achieved by limited biopsy and is usually reliable.

Overproduction of corticotropin by the pituitary gland or extrapituitary tumors leads to hypercortisolism or Cushing syndrome. Diagnosis of suspected Cushing syndrome involves 3 major steps: confirmation of hypercortisolism, differentiation between corticotropin-independent and corticotropin-dependent causes of Cushing syndrome, and distinction between pituitary and ectopic corticotropin production.

A definitive diagnosis of ectopic corticotropin secretion requires stringent criteria, including reversal of the clinical picture after resection of the tumor and/or demonstration of corticotropin immunohistochemical staining within the tumor tissue.

Pulmonary neuroendocrine tumors (pNETs) have distinct pathologic characteristics. Typical carcinoids are indolent neoplasms with a good prognosis, whereas atypical carcinoids have a less indolent behavior. Both are optimally treated with complete surgical excision. More aggressive pNETs often present with local invasion, thoracic lymph nodal metastases, and distant spread. Patients may not be candidates for surgical resection and are treated with chemotherapy and/or radiation therapy. This article examines the potential role of functional imaging evaluation using ^{18}F FDG and somatostatin analogues labeled with ^{68}Ga DOTA-peptides in well-differentiated pNETs with particular attention to clinical and surgical implications.

The aim of this study is to assess in bronchial carcinoid tumors, the prognostic factors in relation to the histology that would determine their most appropriate therapy. The histologic aggressiveness is a determining factor in tumor size and nodal involvement in these tumors. The knowledge of the histologic limits of typical and atypical carcinoid contributes to the recognition of a better valuation of the proportional significance that nodal involvement and histologic grade have in a tumor's prognosis.

Carcinoid tumors are rare lung neoplasms. They may arise centrally or peripherally. For central lesions, bronchoplastic procedures, particularly sleeve resections, are safe and should be the reference for treatment when anatomically and oncologically indicated, independently from pulmonary function.

Large-cell neuroendocrine carcinoma (LCNEC) of the lung is an uncommon aggressive neoplasm with a poor prognosis compared with non–small-cell lung carcinoma (NSCLC). Because of its rarity, the treatment recommendations are not based on clinical trials, but are extrapolated from the approach to patients with NSCLC and small-cell lung carcinoma and the established literature for LCNEC, which is primarily retrospective in nature. Further studies should clarify the histology-specific characteristic and optimal therapeutic approach to establish the entity of LCNEC.

The role of surgery in the management of patients with SCLC remains controversial. Although 2 randomized studies have failed to show any benefit on survival by adding surgery to chemotherapy, retrospective and prospective reports showed that surgery offers a reasonable overall survival in a subset of patients with stage I and II SCLC. Patients' selection is fundamental, and it should include extensive radiologic staging and mediastinal lymph-node biopsy. The use of a PET scan is likely to improve the accuracy of staging. Through primary surgery or after induction chemotherapy, a complete tumor resection associated with systematic lymphadenectomy should be achieved.

Paolo Olivo Lausi, Majed Refai, Pier Luigi Filosso, Enrico Ruffini, Alberto Oliaro, Francesco Guerrera, and Alessandro Brunelli

Thymic neuroendocrine tumors are rare and account for approximately 2% to 5% of all thymic tumors. Despite the suggestion of benign behavior implied by their name, thymic carcinoids have been noted to present a more aggressive biologic behavior than their counterparts in other sites. Because of the lack of data, adequate-sized prospective trials are required for validation, and the enrollment of patients with advanced disease into available clinical trials is encouraged.

Lisa Bodei, Marta Cremonesi, Mark Kidd, Chiara M. Grana, Stefano Severi, Irvin M. Modlin, and Giovanni Paganelli

Peptide receptor radionuclide therapy (PRRT) consists of the systemic administration of a synthetic peptide, labeled with a suitable β-emitting radionuclide, able to irradiate tumors and their metastases via internalization through a specific receptor (usually somatostatin S2), over-expressed on the cell membrane. After almost 2 decades of experience, PRRT, with either ^{90}Y-octreotide or ^{177}Lu-octreotate, has established itself to be an efficient and effective therapeutic modality. As a treatment, it is relatively safe up to the known thresholds of absorbed and bio-effective isotope dosages and the renal and hematological toxicity profiles are acceptable if adequate protective measures are undertaken.

Piero Ferolla

Thoracic Neuroendocrine Tumors (TNETs) range from the more indolent behavior of the well-differentiated to the highly aggressive poorly differentiated forms. A clinical approach totally different in terms of diagnosis and treatment is therefore required. Chemotherapy and radiotherapy are the treatments of choice in poorly differentiated, whereas biological and target therapy, peptide receptor radionuclide therapy (PPRT) and temozolomide have shown efficacy in small series or in the subgroup analysis of larger trials in well differentiated. However, no specific trials have been performed before this year. The first large, prospective, randomized trial (LUNA trial) entirely dedicated to TNET is ongoing at the time of this publication.

THORACIC SURGERY CLINICS

NOW AVAILABLE FOR YOUR iPhone and iPad

Preface

Knowledge of Pulmonary Neuroendocrine Tumors: Where Are We Now?

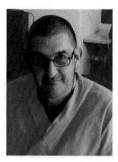

Pier Luigi Filosso, MD, FECTS, FCCP
Editor

Neuroendocrine tumors (NETs) of the lung are regarded as a distinct clinical subgroup of lung cancer, which share particular morphologic, ultrastructural, immunohistochemical, and molecular characteristics. According to the 2004 World Health Organization classification of tumors,[1] they are categorized into 4 major groups,[2] ranging from the low-grade typical carcinoid (TC), to highly aggressive, poorly differentiated tumors (large-cell neuroendocrine carcinoma, LCNC, and small-cell lung cancer, SCLC). Amid them, an intermediate-grade neoplasm (atypical carcinoid, AC) is characterized by a greater aggressive biological behavior, compared to TC with a poorer 5-year survival and a higher tendency to lymph-nodal involvement at presentation. TCs and ACs are categorized together as carcinoids; LCNC is considered a subgroup of large-cell carcinomas, and SCLC is an independent class of lung cancer.

NETs derive from the pulmonary neuroendocrine cells (PNECs), which are of endodermal origin, regardless of their phenotypic resemblance to neurons.[3] In the postnatal phase and later, the PNEC system represents the lung stem cells niche, which is extremely important in the airway epithelial regeneration and carcinogenesis.[4,5] In the healthy adult, the PNECs distribution is quite permeating, with approximately 1 PNEC for every 2500 epithelial cells. Although PNECs are mostly solitary, sometimes they appear aggregate in innervated PNEC clusters, intended as neuroepithelial bodies (NEBs).[6] The precise PNEC biological function remains unclear, as well as that of NEBs. Singular PNEC and NEB have a similar phenotype, because they are the site of adenosine, serotonin, and other amines storage, which play a very important role in normal lung development, growth, and repair. They have been considered to serve as airway chemoreceptors, responsive to hypoxia and thought to activate vagal nerves, participating in breath regulation.[7]

Neuroendocrine cell spread is also thought to be a rare preneoplastic condition: diffuse idiopathic pulmonary neuroendocrine cell hyperplasia (DIPNECH) is, in fact, characterized by a widespread peripheral airway PNEC and NEBs proliferation, while Tumorlet is a nodular neuroendocrine cell proliferation that measures less than 5 mm in diameter. DIPNECHs are also considered a sort of adaptive response in persons that live at high altitudes, as well as a reactive response during lung injuries, the commonest of which are obliterative bronchiolitis and interstitial lung disease, and in patients with chronic cough.[8–10]

Genetic abnormalities have been recently detected and proposed for a better classification of lung NETs. In particular, abnormal expression or loss of heterozygosity and point mutations of the p53 locus on chromosome 17p13 were seen in approximately 4% of TCs, 29% of ACs, and 80%

Thorac Surg Clin 24 (2014) ix–xii
http://dx.doi.org/10.1016/j.thorsurg.2014.05.005
1547-4127/14/$ – see front matter

thoracic.theclinics.com

of LCNCs; this data may support the hypothesis that TC, AC, and LCNC are genetically different from each other.[11,12] Also, the p53 protein frequency was found to be 0% in TCs, 20% in ACs, and 80% in LCNCs, suggesting that this data could be used to better classify these neoplasms.[13]

The recent improvement in histologic diagnostic tools, as well as the rapid diffusion of lung cancer screening programs, resulted in a recent increase in pulmonary NETs recognition; this may explain their rapid growth in incidence, which actually accounts for approximately 30% of all NETs.[14]

Lung NETs comprise roughly 20% of all primary lung cancers; their incidence has been reported to be 1.57/100,000/year, with a median age at presentation of 64 years.

Bronchial carcinoids (both TCs and ACs) have an annual incidence comprised between 2.3 and 2.8 cases/1,000,000 people[15] and include 20% to 25% of all carcinoid tumors, but account for only 3% of all primary lung cancers. Bronchial carcinoids have an equal gender distribution; in the retrospective series, the median age of patients with TC is lower than for those diagnosed with ACs or other neuroendocrine neoplasms.

The majority of TCs are centrally located; whereas ACs and LCNCs tend to be more frequently peripheral, ACs sometimes are greater in size. Despite that patients diagnosed with SCLC and LCNC are likely to have a heavy smoking history, a clear correlation between tobacco exposure and carcinoid development has not yet been demonstrated, even if Fink and colleagues[15] and Filosso and coworkers[16] observed a higher frequency of smokers in their AC group.

Peripheral lesions tend to be asymptomatic, whereas cough, dyspnea, pneumonitis, and hemoptysis are the commonest symptoms in centrally located lesions; in addition, symptoms may be present for many years before the diagnosis, reflecting a possible slow tumor growth.

Paraneoplastic syndromes occur in less than 5% of NETs and are more frequently associated with bronchial carcinoids and SCLCs.

Cushing syndrome, due to an ectopic adrenocorticotropic hormone production and secretion, may occur in less than 2% of carcinoids, whereas less than 1% of patients with Cushing syndrome have a bronchopulmonary carcinoid.

Carcinoid syndrome, characterized by symptoms related to serotonin secretion (diarrhea, wheezing, flushing, and carcinoid heart disease), is very rare (<1% to 3% in bronchial carcinoids) and usually reflects the presence of liver metastases.

The syndrome of inappropriate antidiuretic hormone secretion is the commonest paraneoplastic syndrome in SCLC (approximately 5.5% at the time of diagnosis).[17] It is caused by the antidiuretic hormone disproportionate secretion and is characterized by reduced plasma osmolarity, concentrated urine, and euvolemic hyponatremia.

Less frequent paraneoplastic syndromes include acromegaly, hypercalcemia, hypoglycemia, and myasthenia gravis.

Bronchial carcinoids may also occur as a component (less than 5%) of the familial endocrine cancer syndrome called multiple neuroendocrine neoplasia 1 (MEN1),[18] although the majority occur as sporadic cases. MEN1 is an autosomal-dominant disease, associated with the gene locus on 11q13 and characterized by neoplasms of the pituitary gland, pancreas, and parathyroid.

Surgery is the treatment of choice for bronchial carcinoids; complete tumor resection with preservation of as much lung tissue as possible is to be achieved, whenever feasible. The conservative resection, in the case of TC, could be a sleeve resection (in the case of centrally located lesion), or a segmentectomy or lobectomy. Lobectomy/bilobectomy (depending on the tumor size and its location) may be proposed for AC. Systemic lymphadenectomy[19] must be accomplished in all cases, because lymph nodal metastases are evident in about 40% of ACs.[20]

Surgery achieves a 5- and 10-year survival rate higher than 90% for TCs and 70% and 50%, respectively, for ACs.[20] Recurrences occur in 3% to 5% of TCs, and only 15% of deaths are caused by the tumor, while in ACs the majority of deaths are due to recurrences, which occur in about 26% of cases.

The use of several various chemotherapeutic agents (doxorubicin, 5-fluorouracil, dacarbazine, cisplatin, etoposide, streptozocin, and carboplatin) has been proposed for advanced bronchial carcinoids, but it has yielded minimal and generally short-lasting results.[21] More recently, temozolamide and everolimus have been used, with promising results.

Many LCNCs/SCLCs are poor candidates for surgery, mostly due to their local or systemic spread. Lobectomy and lymphadenectomy are the treatments preferred in early-stage LCNCs, and these procedures may improve survival if no lymph nodal metastases are found. Otherwise, the reported outcome is very poor.[22,23] Recurrences and distant metastases occur early, even after a complete resection and also in stage I tumors[24]; surgery alone does not seem the appropriate treatment and should be followed by chemoradiotherapy.

In SCLC patients with a limited disease (T1-T2 N0), surgery with systemic lymphadenectomy, followed by adjuvant chemoradiotherapy, may be proposed as part of their treatment plan. SCLC is usually extremely sensitive to chemotherapy; the combination of etoposide and cisplatin is most widely used, yielding response rates of 60% to 80%.[25] However, tumor recurrences (or distant metastases) are very common in the first 2 years after the induction treatment.

A great deal of research is needed to better understand the treatment of such rare neoplasms. That is the aim of this publication, which collects papers coming from the most experienced international centers in the scientific community of pathologists, thoracic surgeons, and oncologists.

Two years ago, the European Society of Thoracic Surgeons (www.ests.org) launched a new working group on NETs and a retrospective database was immediately designed. Through this, more than 1900 NETs cases have been collected from several European and American institutions. This database actually represents an important source for future studies and scientific projects, but this is not enough: the next step, in fact, will be the development of a new prospective NETs database, with the aim of collecting the shortest possible time of one of the largest NETs clinical series available for the scientific community. Further efforts by pathologists, biologists, and oncologists are needed to expand the biological behavior of such rare neoplasms, to improve knowledge on their recurrence development mechanisms, as well as on their medical and/or biological treatment. I hope that this publication may serve the scientific community to lead to the development of possible uniform guidelines for NETs management.

I would like to address my special thanks to all the coauthors for their enthusiasm to this project and their strong and valuable effort and expertise in the preparation of their articles. Their help has strongly contributed to improving the quality of this issue of Thoracic Surgery Clinics.

Finally, a special thanks goes to the Elsevier Clinics Department, in particular to Ms Stephanie Carter and Mr John Vassallo: their continuous support and their fantastic professional work greatly facilitate our work.

Pier Luigi Filosso, MD, FECTS, FCCP
Department of Thoracic Surgery
University of Torino
San Giovanni Battista Hospital
Via Genova, 3
Torino 10126, Italy

The European Society of Thoracic Surgeons (ESTS)

Neuroendocrine Tumors of the Lung Working-Group

Steering Committee

Hisao Asamura (Japan)

Alessandro Brunelli (UK)

Pier Luigi Filosso (Italy)

Mariano Garcia-Yuste (Spain)

Eric Lim (UK)

Konstantinos Papagiannopoulos (UK)

Interpal Sarkaria (USA)

Pascal Thomas (France)

E-mail address:
pierluigi.filosso@unito.it

REFERENCES

1. Travis WD, Brambilla E, Mueller-Hermelink HK, et al. Pathology and genetics of tumours of the lung, pleura, thymus and heart. Lyon: IARC Press; 2004.
2. Travis WD. Advances in neuroendocrine lung tumors. Ann Oncol 2010;21:S65–71.
3. Ito T, Nogawa H, Udaka N, et al. Development of pulmonary neuroendocrine cells of fetal hamster in explant culture. Lab Invest 1997;77:449–57.
4. Van Lommel A, Bollé T, Fannes W, et al. The pulmonary neuroendocrine system: the past decade. Arch Histol Cytol 1999;62:1–16.
5. Cutz E, Yeger H, Pan J. Pulmonary neuroendocrine cell system in pediatric lung disease—recent advances. Pediatr Dev Pathol 2007;10:419–35.
6. Lauweryns JM, Van Lommel AT, Dom RJ. Innervation of rabbit intrapulmonary neuroepithelial bodies. Quantitative and qualitative ultrastructural study after vagotomy. J Neurol Sci 1985;67:81–92.
7. Adriaensen D, Brouns I, Pintelon I, et al. Evidence for a role of neuroepithelial bodies as complex airway sensors: comparison with smooth muscle-associated airway receptors. J Appl Physiol 2006; 101:960–70.
8. Irshad S, McLean E, Rankin S, et al. Unilateral diffuse idiopathic pulmonary neuroendocrine cell hyperplasia and multiple carcinoids treated with surgical resection. J Thorac Oncol 2010;5:921–3.
9. Armas OA, White DA, Erlandson RA, et al. Diffuse idiopathic pulmonary neuroendocrine cell proliferation presenting as interstitial lung disease. Am J Surg Pathol 1995;19:963–70.

10. Reyes LJ, Majó J, Perich D, et al. Neuroendocrine cell hyperplasia as an unusual form of interstitial lung disease. Respir Med 2007;101:1840–3.

11. Onuki N, Wistuba II, Travis WD, et al. Genetic changes in the spectrum of neuroendocrine lung tumors. Cancer 1999;85:600–7.

12. Sugio K, Osaki T, Oyama T, et al. Genetic alteration in carcinoid tumors of the lung. Ann Thorac Cardiovasc Surg 2003;9:149–54.

13. Kobayashi Y, Tokuchi Y, Hashimoto T, et al. Molecular markers for reinforcement of histological subclassification of neuroendocrine lung tumors. Cancer Sci 2004;95:334–41.

14. Modlin IM, Lye KD, Kidd M. A 5-decade analysis of 13,715 carcinoid tumors. Cancer 2003;97:934–59.

15. Fink G, Krelbaum T, Yellin A, et al. Pulmonary carcinoid: presentation, diagnosis, and outcome in 142 cases in Israel and review of 640 cases from the literature. Chest 2001;119:1647–51.

16. Filosso PL, Oliaro A, Ruffini E, et al. Outcome and prognostic factors in bronchial carcinoids. A single-center experience. J Thorac Oncol 2013;8:1282–8.

17. Marchioli CC, Graziano SL. Paraneoplastic syndromes associated with small cell lung cancer. Chest Surg Clin N Am 1997;7:65–80.

18. Sachithanandan N, Harle RA, Burgess JR. Bronchopulmonary carcinoid in multiple endocrine neoplasia type 1. Cancer 2005;103:509–15.

19. D'Andrilli A, Venuta F, Rendina EA. The role of lymphadenectomy in lung cancer surgery. Thorac Surg Clin 2012;22:227–37.

20. Detterbeck F. Management of carcinoid tumors. Ann Thorac Surg 2010;89:998–1005.

21. Wirth LJ, Carter MR, Jänne PA, et al. Outcome of patients with pulmonary carcinoid tumors receiving chemotherapy or chemoradiotherapy. Lung Cancer 2004;44:213–20.

22. Lim E, Yap YK, De Stavola BL, et al. The impact of stage and cell type on the prognosis of pulmonary neuroendocrine tumors. J Thorac Cardiovasc Surg 2005;130:969–72.

23. Filosso PL, Ruffini E, Di Gangi S, et al. Prognostic factors in neuroendocrine tumours of the lung: a single-centre experience. Eur J Cardiothorac Surg 2014;45(3):521–6.

24. Veronesi G, Morandi U, Alloisio M, et al. Large cell neuroendocrine carcinoma of the lung: a retrospective analysis of 144 surgical cases. Lung Cancer 2006;53:111–5.

25. Noda K, Nishiwaki Y, Kawahara M, et al. Irinotecan plus cisplatin compared with etoposide plus cisplatin for extensive small-cell lung cancer. N Engl J Med 2002;346:85–91.

A Historical Appreciation of Bronchopulmonary Neuroendocrine Neoplasia
Resolution of a Carcinoid Conundrum

Irvin M. Modlin, MD, PhD, DSc, MA, FRCS (Eng. & Ed), FCS (SA)[a,b,]*,
Lisa Bodei, MD, PhD[c], Mark Kidd, PhD[a]

KEYWORDS

- Atypical carcinoid • APUD • Azzopardi • Bronchial adenoma • Bronchopulmonary carcinoid
- Capella • Carcinoid • Chevalier Jackson

KEY POINTS

- In the three-quarters of a century that have elapsed since the first description of a bronchial carcinoid, the field has progressed from serendipitous radiological or bronchoscopic diagnosis to computed tomography, magnetic resonance imaging, and somatostatin receptor imaging identification. Similarly, pathologic techniques have advanced from a naïve assessment of neoplasia to a delineation of several tumor subtypes and an understanding of the neuroendocrine basis of the disease process.
- Endoscopic therapy has evolved from bronchoscopic resection to laser ablation and surgical ablation from sleeve resection to lobectomy and lymph node clearance.
- The recent usage of somatostatin receptor targeted Lutetium-177 or Yttrium-90 peptide receptor radiotherapy to treat residual disease or metastases represents the full turn of the circle because radiation, which initiated diagnosis at the turn of the nineteenth century, has now, a century later, become the novel therapeutic strategy.
- Current pathologic analyses are limited in their ability to precisely define the malignancy of a lesion and predict the likelihood of recurrence.
- The issues of the future that remain to be resolved are early detection of tumors by molecular blood biomarkers, establishment of the individual genomic tumor patterns that define the biologic behavior of each tumor, and the identification of the tumor interactome and master regulators that will precisely facilitate targeted therapy.
- A key unresolved question is the identification of the genetic and environmental activators that are responsible for the initiation of pulmonary neuroendocrine cell proliferation and neoplastic transformation.

FROM GNOSIS TO SUNESIS

In the eighteenth and nineteenth centuries, lung disease was difficult to diagnose and even more difficult to treat. Visualization of the lung was only possible postmortem and operative intervention was impossible in the absence of anesthesia and positive pressure ventilation. The stethoscope

The authors have nothing to disclose.
[a] Department of Surgery, Yale School of Medicine, 310 Cedar Street, New Haven, CT 06520, USA; [b] Wren Laboratories, Branford, CT 06405, USA; [c] Division of Nuclear Medicine, European Institute of Oncology, via Ripamonti 435, Milan 20141, Italy
* Corresponding author. Department of Surgery, Yale School of Medicine, 310 Cedar Street, New Haven, CT 06520.
E-mail address: imodlin@optonline.net

thoracic.theclinics.com

described by Laennec (1781–1826) in 1816 had replaced the percussive technique of Auenbrugger (1722–1809) as a clinical tool but neither yielded great insight into pulmonary pathology (**Fig. 1**). Diseases of the chest were for the most part infectious and tuberculosis (TB) remained the scourge of the time as the most prevalent cause of lung pathologic abnormality. Almost all knowledge was gleaned from the extensive autopsy series of Rokitansky (1804–1878), but minimal clinical diagnostic tools were available other than visual

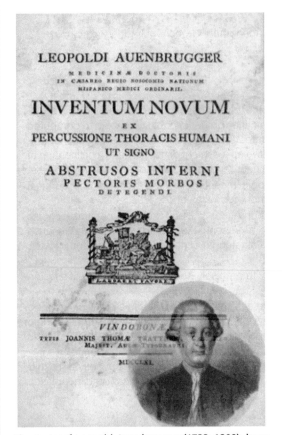

Fig. 1. Josef Leopold Auenbrugger (1722–1809), born in Graz, invented percussion as a diagnostic technique. This skill was initially acquired in testing the level of wine casks in the cellar of his father's hotel but was translated into the first diagnostic test for pulmonary disease. His published text, *Inventum Novum ex Percussione Thoracis Humani Interni Pectoris Morbos Detegendi* (*A New Discovery that Enables the Physician from the Percussion of the Human Thorax to Detect the Diseases Hidden Within the Chest*) has been regarded as a book that defines a new epoch in the modern history of medicine. Auenbrugger's method of diagnosis at first met with indifference but was noted by the French physician René Laennec (1781–1826), who, pursuing a similar train of thought, thereafter developed the technique of auscultation. (*Courtesy of Irvin M. Modlin, MD, New Haven, CT.*)

examination of the sputum. Given the low life expectancy and the limitations of hygiene and ventilation, infections and TB were the dominant pulmonary diseases. By the end of the nineteenth century, tumors of the lung were considered a rarity, although attention was focused on them as observant physicians began to note their relationship to inhaled agents, such as radon, asbestos, tobacco, and silica, based on industrial exposure. The advent of radiology and bronchoscopy at the beginning of the twentieth century combined with the advance of histology dramatically amplified the ability to diagnose pulmonary disease, identify tumors, and begin to characterize them. Thus, lung neoplasia became a source of increasing clinical focus as public health techniques improved TB management and the disease focus began to shift. The consideration of lung cancer as a rare disease in the first decade of the twentieth century had dramatically shifted by the mid-century to a realization of its major clinical impact. A further issue was the evolving understanding that such tumors were substantially different in clinical behavior and could be differentiated by their histopathological patterns. Although most attention was focused on the highly aggressive squamous and adenocarcinoma variants, it became apparent that a subset of tumors initially designated bronchial adenomas behaved differently and required reassessment. The elucidation of the neuroendocrine cell system and the description by Oberndorfer (1876–1944) of a gastrointestinal tumor termed, *Karzinoide* (1907), led to the recognition that such lesions might have a pulmonary equivalent.

Armed with this knowledge, pathologists addressed the question of identifying and categorizing such tumors to best inform clinicians, in particular surgeons, as to the optimal management of pulmonary carcinoid tumors. The crux of the matter related to the delineation of specific pulmonary neuroendocrine tumor subtypes, each of which carried a substantially different prognosis and therefore required a significantly different management strategy. This article documents the evolution of the understanding of bronchopulmonary neuroendocrine tumor disease and the elucidation of the stratagems that have led to the current understanding of its genesis and management.

EARLY OBSERVATIONS ON LUNG TUMORS

Early literature indicates that the first description of a neoplastic lesion of the lung emanates from Morgagni (1682–1771), who in 1761, described an *ulcus cancrosum* of the right lung in an autopsy on a 60-year-old man (**Fig. 2**).[1] In 1821, Andral[2] suggested that examination of the color of sputum

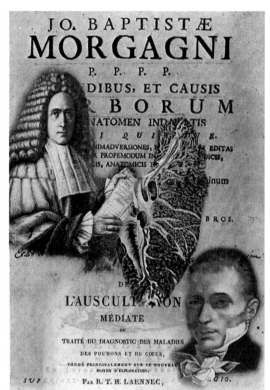

Fig. 2. Giovanni Battista Morgagni (1682–1771) (*top left*), an Italian anatomist, educated in Bologna and subsequently the chair of Theoretical Medicine in Padua, is regarded as the father of modern anatomic pathology. His text of 1761, *De Sedibus et Causis Morborum per Anatomem Indagatis,* provided a complete integration of pathologic findings and their correlation with clinical findings of 646 patients, including a lung tumor. René-Théophile-Hyacinthe Laennec (*bottom right*) (1781–1826), of Quimper, France, invented the stethoscope in 1816, while working at the Hôpital Necker. The mode of discovery is of interest. Unable to use percussion to diagnose an obese woman's heart, complaint Laennec wrote, "*I rolled a quire of paper into a kind of cylinder and applied one end of it to the region of the heart and the other to my ear, and was not a little surprised and pleased to find that I could thereby perceive the action of the heart in a manner much more clear and distinct than I had ever been able to do by the immediate application of my ear.*" Ironically, he perished of TB (*center*) after a brief Professorship at the Collège de France. Not all physicians accepted the new stethoscope. Although the *New England Journal of Medicine* reported the invention of the stethoscope in 1821, as late as 1885, a professor of medicine stated, "*He that hath ears to hear, let him use his ears and not a stethoscope.*" Thus, the founder of the American Heart Association, L. A. Connor (1866–1950), carried a silk handkerchief with him to place on the wall of the chest for ear auscultation. (*Courtesy of Irvin M. Modlin, MD, New Haven, CT.*)

could facilitate diagnosis of lung lesions; he associated green sputum with blood and lung disease. It was, however, Laennec's description of an unusual lung mass, a "crude yellow tubercle," in 1831[3] that probably represents the first description of a bronchial carcinoid.

His subsequent description of the stethoscope provided the basis for scientific diagnosis of lung disease, but there are no reports of its specific usage for identification of lung tumors. By 1846, Bell (cited in Ref.[4]) had opined on the condition of lung tumors and outlined a strategy for diagnosis, the likelihood of which was pointed out in terms of environmental influence by the 1879 report of Harting and Hesse,[5] who described the increased incidence in radon miners in Schneeberg. These lung tumors were designated lymphosarcoma and, as such, proved to be a seminal observation in establishing that lung tumors were not only related to inhaled agents, but that such lesions might represent different pathologic entities. The former observation was confirmed by Rottman[6] in 1898 in his description of lung cancers in Leipzig tobacco workers. Nevertheless, lung tumors per se were still regarded as rare and when Adler, in 1912, published a book entitled, *Primary Malignant Growths of the Lungs and Bronchi,*[4] he reported all cases of lung cancer in the published literature worldwide and could verify only 374 cases.

DIAGNOSIS OF LUNG NEUROENDOCRINE TUMORS
Radiology

The precise localization of lung tumors was greatly facilitated at the turn of the nineteenth century by the advent of the new discipline of radiology. In May 1897, Williams[7] of Boston at the meeting of the Association of American Physicians provided an early comprehensive discussion of the use of radiographs in thoracic diseases, including pulmonary TB, pneumonia, and pleural effusions. He particularly stressed the correlation of radiographic appearances with the pathologic findings, which he corroborated by postmortem examination. Given the relative unawareness of lung cancers, early radiologists were most concerned with TB, and even early instruments were able to identify tubercles the size of a pinhead. Although Frankel had earlier noted that radiographs were of little service in the diagnosis of lung tumors, Adler,[4] in 1912, concluded that improvements in technology had facilitated the diagnosis of mass lesions. Thus, by 1917, McMahon and Carman[8] had described in detail the radiographic appearance of primary carcinomas of the lungs and offered differential points in distinguishing these rare tumors from other intrathoracic conditions. By 1918, pulmonary metastases were identifiable and, in 1919, Pfahler reported that metastatic disease of the lungs was common and, although recognizable, was not definable by radiograph.

Jackson[9] reported the installation of bismuth subcarbonate into the bronchial tree to identify foreign bodies in 1918, while Sicard and Forestier,[10] in 1924, used lipiodol to facilitate the identification of bronchial or peribronchial masses. The use of transthoracic needle aspiration biopsy for the diagnosis of cancer was described in the early 1930s by Martin and Ellis.[11] In Kerley's address to the First International Congress of Radiology in 1925,[12] he included 2 radiograph images of bronchial carcinoma. Thereafter, in 1936, Peterson[13] published on the "bizarre, but characteristic lobar atelectasis" in benign bronchial adenomas. Within 10 years, Allen, in 1946,[14] reported a bronchial adenoma in a 36-year-old woman demonstrating a circular opacity on the right side, which was posteriorly situated, with an area of atelectasis distal to it. Two years later, a mass radiography campaign in Edinburgh identified 71 patients (of 300,000) with bronchial carcinoma: 2 additional patients had "bronchial adenoma" (cited in Ref.[15]). In 1964, Hattori and coworkers[16] were the first to describe the use of metal and nylon bronchial pressures to diagnose carcinoma nodules using fluoroscopically guided preformed transnasal catheters. The accuracy was even further improved by Dahlgren,[17] who, in 1966, described fluoroscopically guided fine needle aspiration.

Bronchoscopy

In 1898, Killian[18] was the first to popularize the use of a bronchoscope to directly visualize lesions, and 2 years thereafter, used the device to remove a foreign body. Subsequently, Jackson[19] (1865–1965) of Philadelphia, in 1914, reported the first bronchoscopic resection of a lung tumor, presumably a bronchial adenoma (**Fig. 3**). The technique remained more an art than science until Broyles introduced the telescope optic for bronchoscopy in Baltimore in 1940, followed by the optical forceps (1948), thereby facilitating not only visualization but biopsy and histologic assessment. Hopkins,[20] in 1954, then introduced a rod-lens telescope system that considerably improved the lighting and imaging through the rigid bronchoscope. Subsequently, Ikeda (1962) developed the flexible fiberscope using glass fiber illumination for the rigid bronchoscope. This technology was adopted by Storz as a cold light illumination source for his rigid bronchoscopes in 1963 and thereby facilitated identification and resection of

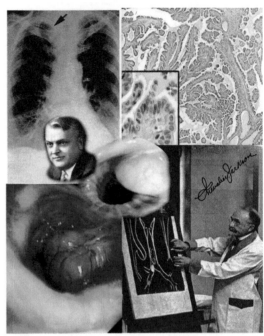

Fig. 3. Russell Carman (1875–1826) (*top left*) of the Mayo Clinic was a pioneer in the early use of radiology and described the appearance of bronchial adenomas (*arrowhead*). Chevalier Jackson (1865–1958) of Philadelphia, known as the father of endoscopy, first identified and resected bronchial adenomas (*bottom left and center*) using a rigid bronchoscope. Early histologic descriptions relied on H&E staining (*top right*) to demonstrate their "carcinoid" origin. (*Courtesy of* Irvin M. Modlin, MD, New Haven, CT.)

bronchial adenomas by biopsy.[21] In 1912, Davies[22] (1879–1965) undertook a lobectomy to successfully resect a bronchial carcinoma (**Table 1**).

Histopathology

Lung tumors were initially diagnosed at autopsy and descriptive terminology did not allow for the delineation of different lesions. Tumors were therefore variously characterized as cicatrizing, scirrhous, or ulcerating, and many presumably were advanced forms of TB misdiagnosed as neoplasia. The classical descriptions of morbid pathologic abnormality provided by Rokitansky were replaced by the era of Virchow and the advent of cellular histopathology.

In this respect, the contributions of early pathologists such as Kulchitsky (1856–1925), Oberndorfer, Masson (1880–1959), Hamperl (1899–1976), and Froelich led to the recognition that not only were specialized cells (chromaffin) involved but their proliferation into tumors provided a basis for understanding the pathogenesis of the lesions (**Fig. 4**).

Table 1
Historical timeline of the elucidation of pulmonary NET

Author, Date	Observations
Morgagni,[1] 1761	Description of lung cancer: *ulcus cancrosum* identified at autopsy in the right lung of a 60-year-old man
Andral,[2] 1821	Description of the use of sputum to diagnose lung cancer
Laennec,[3] 1831	Description of an intrabronchial mass
Bell,[4] 1846	Diagnosis of a primary lung tumor
Harting & Hesse,[5] 1879	High frequency of "lymphosarcoma" (lung cancer) in autopsied miners in Schneeberg (*Schneeberger Lungenkrebs*), Silesia (Radon exposure)
Killian,[18] 1898	First bronchoscopy
Rottmann,[6] 1898	Lung cancer in Leipzig tobacco workers—dust inhalation
Adler,[4] 1912	Noted rarity of lung cancer and that the disease occurs disproportionately in men and in the right lung
Davies,[22] 1913	Lobectomy for a primary bronchial carcinoma
Jackson,[19] 1914	First bronchoscopic resection of a large intrabronchial tumor
Barnard,[27] 1926	Histologic identification of an "oat-celled sarcoma of the mediastinum"—small-cell lung carcinoma (SCLC)
Geipel,[29] 1931	Identification of bronchial lesions, "Basalzellkrebs"
Graham et al,[90] 1933	First surgical removal of an entire lung (carcinoma of the bronchus)
Gloyme,[91] 1936	"Oat-cell carcinoma" of the lung and asbestos exposure
Hamperl,[30] 1937	First identification of a bronchial carcinoid
Clara,[70] 1937	Identification of pluripotential progenitor cells in lung
Eloesser,[92] 1939	First bronchotomy for resection of a bronchial tumor
Holley,[38] 1946	Identified one case with argentaffin granules in a series of 30 bronchial adenomas
Froelich,[67] 1949	Described the presence of clear cells "Helle Zelle" in the bronchial mucosa—arranged either singly or in corpuscular aggregates "*Knoetchen*." Proposed a neuroectodermal origin and a chemoreceptive function
Liebow,[42] 1952	Referred to minute epithelial lesions (later associated with "tumorlets") as "carcinoid atypical proliferation"
Biorck et al,[46] 1952	First report of carcinoid syndrome and its relation to a metastatic carcinoid tumor
Prior,[93] 1953	Recognized that the "unusual" epithelial hyperplasia (later considered "tumorlets") in minute peripheral lung tumors closely resembled the structure of the carcinoid type of bronchial adenoma
Felton,[94] 1953	Description of minute adenomas in the bronchioles (away from the mucous glands). Proposed an epithelial origin
Whitwell,[95] 1954	Devised the term "tumorlet" (a minute epithelia lesion) and considered their formation a response to tissue injury
Price-Thomas,[96] 1955	Sleeve resection of the bronchus stem
Feyrter,[39] 1956	Confirmed existence of *Helle Zelle* cells in the lung and included them in the DNES classification
Kincaid-Smith & Brossy,[49] 1956	Reported a case of carcinoid syndrome 6 y after lobectomy for a bronchial adenoma, the symptoms produced by hepatic metastases
Stanford et al,[50] 1958	Carcinoid syndrome in association with a bronchial carcinoid
Azzopardi,[33] 1959	Histologic identification of SCLC, relationship to carcinoid
Pearse et al,[24,53] 1960's	Development of APUD doctrine and delineation of "oat-cell tumors" as a component of the "neurocrestopathies"

(continued on next page)

Table 1
(continued)

Author, Date	Observations
Bensch et al,[97] 1965	Demonstration of Kulchitsky cells in normal bronchial glands. Proposed them as the dominant component of carcinoid tumors arising in larger bronchi
Gmelich et al,[71] 1967	Reanalysis of Felton's samples (1953) identified intracytoplasmic spherical granules identical to the neurosecretory granules of the Kulchitsky cells
Baldwin & Grimes,[98] 1967	Described 2 types of bronchial (adenoma) tumor as "benign" and "malignant" carcinoid
Bensch et al,[34] 1968	Identified that pulmonary carcinoid and oat-cell carcinomas were part of a spectrum of neuroendocrine neoplasia. Included SCLC in the APUDoma group of tumors
Lauweryns & Peuskens,[68] 1972	Description of Froelich's bronchial clear cell aggregates and termed them NEBs, which they had originally identified in the lungs of infants in 1969
Arrigoni et al,[75] 1972	Identified "atypical" more aggressive lung carcinoids
Bergsagel et al,[99] 1972	SCLC treated with a combination of thoracic radiation and chemotherapy
Churg & Warnock,[100] 1976	Identified tumorlets in bronchiectasis/emphysema and concluded they were minute peripheral carcinoids
Bonikos et al,[72] 1976	Working with Bensch confirmed the relationship between carcinoids and tumorlets
Godwin & Brown,[101] 1977	Identified contrasting epidemiology for carcinoids and SCLC in terms of age, sex, and smoking history
Ranchod,[102] 1977	Identified the histogenesis of tumorlet: carcinoid lesions noting a connective tissue response (fibrosis on invasion)
Ranchod & Levine,[73] 1980	Spindle cell peripheral pulmonary carcinoid tumors—suggested association between neuroendocrine hyperplasia, tumorlets, and peripheral carcinoids
Gould et al,[103] 1983	Injury-induced hyperplasia of lung NEBs and NE cells
Gould et al,[63] 1983	First classification of BPC
Gould et al,[63] 1983; Warren et al,[64] 1984	Evidence for multiple hormone production in lung carcinoids
Hammond & Sause,[81] 1985	Immunohistochemical identification of large-cell undifferentiated carcinomas, with neuroendocrine differentiation
Warren et al,[82] 1985	Four-stage classification of lung NECs proposed: typical carcinoids, well-differentiated NECs, intermediate NECs, and SCLCs
Aguayo et al,[77] 1992	Description of diffuse hyperplasia and dysplasia of pulmonary NE cells, multiple carcinoid tumorlets, and peribronchiolar fibrosis obliterating small airways. Introduced the term "DIPNECH"
Maini et al,[104] 1993	Isotopic identification of somatostatin receptor expression. Nuclear medicine diagnosis, Octreoscan (SCLC)
Iser et al,[105] 1994	Localization of a bronchial carcinoid by Octreoscan
Armas et al,[78] 1995	Diffuse pulmonary endocrine cell hyperplasia with alveolar space nodules
Travis et al,[87] 1998	Clinicopathological classification spectrum proposed including large-cell lung cancer, large-cell NECs, SCLCs, and NETs
Travis et al,[89] 2004	WHO-based tumor classification

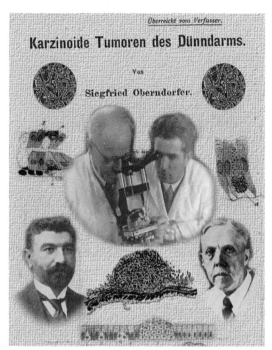

Fig. 4. Siegfried Oberndorfer (1876–1944) (*center*) of the Pathological Institute of the University of Munich was the first to characterize (in 1907) the nature of the "karzinoide" ("carcinoma-like") tumors of the small bowel (*dunndarm*) and refer to them as "benign carcinomas." In 1929, he amended his classification to include the possibility that these small bowel tumors could be malignant and also metastasize. In 1914, using silver impregnation techniques, Pierre Masson (1880–1959) (*bottom left*) and Andre Gosset (1872–1944) (*bottom right*) demonstrated that carcinoid tumors might arise from enterochromaffin cells (Kulchitsky cells) within the glands of Lieberkühn. In 1928, Masson characterized carcinoids as argentaffin cell tumors. (*Courtesy of* Irvin M. Modlin, MD, New Haven, CT.)

The description by Feyrter (1895–1973) of a diffuse syncytium of neuroendocrine cells (NEC) distributed throughout the body (diffuse neuroendocrine system, DNES), including the lungs, allowed for the recognition of the neuroendocrine basis of bronchopulmonary neuroendocrine tumors (BPNETs). In particular, it enabled a distinction to be drawn between "carcinoid" tumors and adenosquamous- and squamous lung cancers. The advent of sophisticated immunohistochemical stains by Grimelius that identified argyrophilic/argentaffin cells,[23] amine precursor uptake and decarboxylases (APUD) by Pearse (1916–2003),[24] and specific peptide and amine products (Polak)[25] further facilitated the distinction of individual types of BPNETs.[26]

As familiarity with lung cancer increased, it became apparent that the initial pathologic thoughts of the nature of such tumors required

substantial reconsideration as the science of histology evolved and techniques for more subtle appreciation of different cancer types became available. In this respect, the description of the entities of squamous carcinoma, adenocarcinomas, and variants including oat-cell tumors and small cell cancers were also evolving during the first half of the twentieth century. In 1926, a hitherto unreported small-cell tumor ("oat-celled sarcoma") of the mediastinum was reported by Barnard,[27] although the term "oat-cell carcinoma" of the lung was initially used in a brief report on asbestos exposure in 1936. The first major paper on this different lung cancer, "oat-cell carcinoma," was written by McKeown[28] of Belfast, Ireland, in 1952. The issue of pathologic tumor types, however, became convoluted and complex as both Liebow (1911–1978) of Yale University and McKeown acknowledged that such malignant neoplasms had been previously reported in the lung and other sites as "oat-cell sarcoma," "round-cell sarcoma," "small-cell carcinoma," "anaplastic-cell carcinoma," or "spindle-cell carcinoma." Thereafter, the concept emerged that there existed a spectrum in cellular composition of oat-cell carcinomas that included other tumors that had previously been referred to using a variety of terminologies. Thus, as early as 1931, Geipel[29] (1869–1956) (better known for the Aschoff-Geipel bodies, microscopically identifiable myocardial granuloma consequent on rheumatic fever), a pathologist from Dresden, had described a separate entity that he referred to as a bronchial *Basalzellkrebs*. This term referred to the entity "bronchial adenomata" and thereby raised the possibility of yet another pathologic lesion different from previously described histologic lung tumor types.

Hamperl,[30] in 1937, at the Charité in Berlin was, however, the first to clearly recognize the true nature of these tumors as carcinoids and is therefore considered to have primacy in correctly categorizing these lesions as bronchial carcinoids (**Fig. 5**). His observations reflected the emerging consensus that the enterochromaffin cells initially described in the gut by Heidenhein (1834–1897) and further adumbrated on by Kulchitsky and Ciaccio (1877–1956) were present in every organ and tissue.[31] Hamperl's prescient observations reflected his knowledge of the original descriptions of a novel form of small bowel tumor described by Oberndorfer[32] of Munich and alluded to by the term "*Karzinoide*."

Thereafter, pathologists and laboratory scientists began to report pulmonary tumors comprised completely of these enterochromaffin cells or lesions whereby such cells were also evident as a component of the tumor. Thus, for a period of

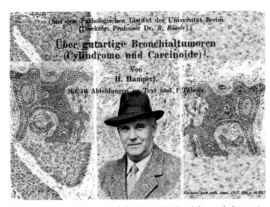

Fig. 5. Herwig Hamperl (1899–1976), although born in Vienna, worked variously in Prague, Berlin, Moscow, Marburg, and Bonn. Although bronchial adenoma was first recognized at necropsy in 1882 by Muller, similar cases were reported by Heine (1927) and Reisner (1928). In 1930, Kramer was the first to clinically diagnose the lesion and note that it might become malignant. Clerf and Crawford (1936) described the tumor as benign and arising from the mucous glands of the bronchus. In 1937, Hamperl, while at the Charité in Berlin, described the entity of bronchial adenoma as comprising 2 pathologic variants, namely, cylindroid and carcinoid. He maintained that the carcinoid variety of bronchial adenoma, unlike the carcinoid tumor of the *appendix vermiformis*, did not contain argentaffin cells. This observation subsequently proved to be invalid (Holley, 1946; Feyrter, 1959; Williams and Azzopardi, 1960). (*Courtesy of* Irvin M. Modlin, MD, New Haven, CT.)

time, some degree of confusion existed between what were considered variants of oat-cell carcinoma or lesions representing the carcinoid entity. The ill-understood issue of carcinoids would, however, remain a controversial area for many years until 1959, when the histopathologist, Azzopardi[33] (1929–2013), reported the characteristic overlapping of crushed nuclei and bluish discoloration of the wall of capillary vessels in oat-cell carcinomas (**Fig. 6**). Thus, by the 1960s, it became established that the histogenesis of oat-cell carcinoma was distinctly different from that of other pulmonary carcinomas. This situation was further clarified in 1968, by Bensch of Yale, who recognized that oat-cell carcinoma and carcinoid tumors were histogenetically related.[34] Nevertheless, there existed for some time an acceptance that typical well-differentiated carcinoid represented one end of the spectrum and the typical small-cell (oat-cell) carcinoma represented the other end of the spectrum of neoplastic lung lesions. In this concept, it was proposed that the atypical or intermediate forms were the link between the typical forms and that, by the 1980s, this notion became widely accepted. Furthermore, as a consequence

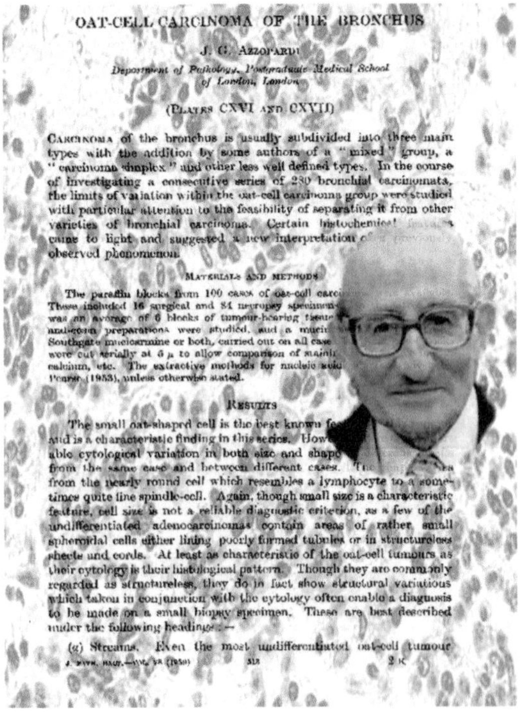

Fig. 6. John Azzopardi (1929–2013), of the Hammersmith Hospital, London. In 1959, his description of the epithelial histogenesis of bronchial oat-cell carcinoma allowed it to be distinguished from anaplastic adenocarcinoma and squamous cell carcinoma. In addition to identifying the 6 distinct features of SCLC, Azzopardi also described variants, including pseudorosettes, ribbons and festoons, and spindle and insular patterns, which were all histologically similar to carcinoids. These observations of neuroendocrine features led him to similar observations of neuroendocrine (divergent) differentiation associated with gastric, cervical, prostatic, and breast carcinomas. Apart from his contributions to pulmonary pathology, he described the pathology of "nonendocrine tumors" associated with Cushing syndrome and paraneoplastic syndromes. (*Courtesy of* Irvin M. Modlin, MD, New Haven, CT.)

of the overlapping microscopic appearance of carcinoids and small-cell (oat-cell) carcinomas, pathologists tended to over-diagnose carcinoids as small-cell (oat-cell) carcinoma.

BRONCHIAL ADENOMAS

Although a bronchial adenoma was initially recognized at the necropsy of a woman who suffered from hemoptysis and chronic cough by Muller in 1882,[35] it was Heine,[36] in 1927, who documented the first series of these tumors. In 1930, Kramer[37] became the first to clinically diagnose the condition and noted that although these were slow growing, in general, there existed a propensity in some for malignant change. This finding encapsulated the prevailing concept that bronchial adenomas were benign, circumscribed glandular tumors of mucosal origin (polypoid or sessile) that were located in the proximal bronchi and therefore substantially different, by virtue of localization, rate of growth, and low level of malignancy, from bronchogenic carcinoma. Hamperl,[30] in 1937, distinguished for the first time the existence of 2 varieties of bronchial adenoma, which he described as either cylindroid or carcinoid in nature. He erroneously considered that bronchial carcinoids, unlike gastrointestinal carcinoids, did not contain argentaffin cells. In 1946, Holley[38] corrected this oversight and was further supported in his views by Feyrter (1959)[39] and Williams and Azzopardi (1960).[40]

Indeed, the subsequent inclusion of bronchial adenomas of carcinoid phenotype as foregut tumors by Williams and Sandler[41] in their carcinoid classification scheme (1963) axiomatically accepted the presence of functional NEC in the tumors (**Fig. 7**). In the intervening time, Liebow[42] had further subdivided the pathologic abnormality of bronchial adenomas to include carcinoids, cylindromas, and mucoepidermoid tumors. He considered the mucoepidermoid tumors as having arisen from bronchial mucous glands, to be mucus secreting, and to exhibit a close resemblance to mixed salivary gland tumors (**Fig. 8**). The cylindromas were described as similar to carcinoids but capable of extension along the bronchial wall, with areas of irregular protrusion firmer. Cylindroma consisted of branching acini, often lined with 2 layers, whereas the acinar lumina may be traversed by cellular bridges. Large tongue-like protrusions of cell masses were noted and the acini described as often full of mucicarmine-positive acidophilic granular material. Cylindromas were less vascular and more prone to invade cartilage, septi, and parenchyma than carcinoid tumors.

Although Logan as early as 1948 had noted the likelihood of malignancy in adenomas, until the 1960s, bronchial adenomas were considered to be uniformly benign lesions and were treated by bronchoscopic excision. Thereafter, several authors, including Goodner,[43] Weiss,[44] and Zellos[15] opined that some lesions exhibited local invasion as well as a potential for metastatic spread. They therefore proposed that bronchial adenomas be reclassified as potentially malignant tumors. The overall clinical thesis was that, although such tumors might exhibit a slower rate of growth and be less likely to metastasize than bronchogenic carcinoma, a more radical approach was indicated than simple resection as for a benign adenoma.

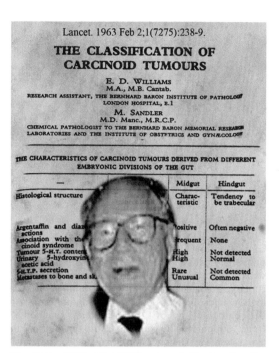

Fig. 7. In 1963, E.D. Williams and Merton Sandler (*bottom*) classified "carcinoid" tumors based on their presumed embryonic site of origin (*background*). This classification system distinguished between NET arising in the foregut (bronchopulmonary, stomach, duodenum, biliary tree, pancreas), midgut (small intestine, appendix, right colon, ovary, testis), and hindgut (transverse colon, left colon, rectum). The criteria for classification included histology (silver staining), serotonin (5-HTP) production, and its product 5-HIAA as well as symptoms consistent with the "carcinoid syndrome." Bronchopulmonary NETs are not usually argentaffinophylic and some produce low levels of serotonin. (*Courtesy of* Irvin M. Modlin, MD, New Haven, CT.)

CARCINOID TUMORS AND THE DIFFUSE NEUROENDOCRINE SYSTEM

In the nineteenth century, Langhans (1839–1915), Lubarsch (1860–1933), and Ransom (1860–1909) described unusual tumors in the small bowel but each failed to adequately investigate these novel entities (**Fig. 9**).[31] This responsibility fell to Oberndorfer, who became the first to adequately characterize the nature of the lesions and refer to them as "benign carcinomas." During his tenure at the Pathologic Institute of the University of Munich, Oberndorfer[32] noted that these tumors were distinct clinical entities and named them "karzinoide" ("carcinoma-like"), emphasizing their benign features. The recognition of carcinoids as endocrine-related tumors was first outlined by Gosset and Masson in 1914.[45] Two decades later, in 1929, Oberndorfer amended his original

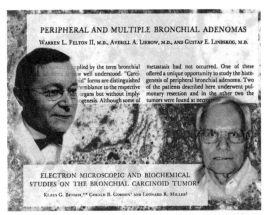

Fig. 8. Averill Liebow (1911–1978) (*left*) of Yale is considered one of the founding fathers of modern pulmonary pathology and was involved in a series of seminal studies ranging from the anatomy of bronchopulmonary circulation and musculature to the identification of lung lesions and adumbrations on the pathobiology of "bronchogenic carcinoma" (*top*). Supported by grants from the Office of Naval Research, Liebow established a research laboratory in cardiopulmonary disease. Klaus Bensch (*bottom right*) was invited by Liebow to work with him to study the nature of the Kulchitsky cell in the lung. His electron-micrographic work (*bottom*) helped to establish the endocrine nature of the lesions and allowed for the subsequent development of a series of classification systems based on a "neuroendocrine spectrum" for this disease. (*Courtesy of* Irvin M. Modlin, MD, New Haven, CT.)

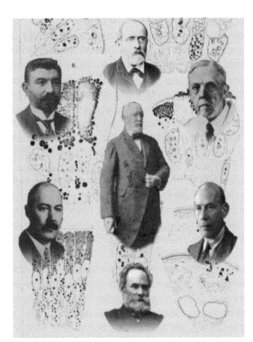

Fig. 9. Nikolai Kulchitsky (1856–1925) (*center*) of Kharkov University described, in 1897, a unique type of cell of the intestinal epithelium that subsequently became widely referred to as the Kulchitsky cell. This cell type is currently referred to as the enterochromaffin cell based on the 1906 observations of Carmèlo Ciaccio (1877–1956) (*bottom right*), who proposed that the intestinal crypt cells be referred to as "enterochromaffin" given their propensity to staining with chromium salts. Pierre Masson (1880–1959) (*top left*) developed the eponymous trichrome stain and, in 1914, with Andre Gosset (1872–1944) (*top right*) demonstrated the argentaffin staining properties of neuroendocrine tumor cells. They suggested that the Kulchitsky cell formed a diffuse endocrine organ. Such a concept was later more fully developed by Freiderich Feyrter (1895–1973) (*bottom left*), who developed the DNES concept based on his recognition of argyrophil and argentaffin cells in the prostate gland, urethra, urinary bladder, and Littre glands as well as in the lung system. All these cell-based observations were predicated on the work of Rudolf Heidenhain (1834–1897) (*top*), who first identified human gastrointestinal tract NEC, whereas the concept of a diffuse neural and endocrine regulatory system was based on the work of Ivan P. Pavlov (1848–1936) (*bottom*), who was awarded a Nobel Prize in 1904 for research on the neural regulation of digestive activity. Abnormalities in the neural regulation of the lung are considered one of the mechanisms for the pathogenesis of bronchopulmonary complications including fibrotic and autoimmune processes. (*Courtesy of* Irvin M. Modlin, MD, New Haven, CT.)

classification to include the possibility that these small bowel tumors could be malignant and also metastasize. Although the enterochromaffin cell, the carcinoid cell of origin, had been identified as early as 1897 by Kulchitsky, it was not until 1953 that Lembeck established that such cells synthesized and secreted serotonin, a potent bioactive amine. Thereafter, the protean clinical effects of serotonin, including "flushing," were recognized as were the associated relationship of carcinoid heart disease (1952; Biork and colleagues[46]) and fibrosis (1961; Moertel and colleagues[47]). In 1963, Williams and Sandler[41] classified carcinoids according to their embryologic site of origin as foregut carcinoids (respiratory tract, stomach, duodenum, biliary system, and pancreas), midgut carcinoids (small intestine, appendix, cecum, and proximal colon), and hindgut carcinoids (distal colon and rectum).[41] This classification was the first to emphasize clinicopathological differences between the tumor groups comprising the gastroenteropancreatic neuroendocrine tumors (GEP-NETs) but never achieved general acceptance in routine diagnostic practice, as it proved too imprecise to distinguish between the different

biologically relevant GEP-NET entities. This lack of precision was particularly apparent in the foregut NETs, which included bronchopulmonary carcinoids, because they differ so greatly in morphology, function, and biology that they proved impossible to classify within a single group, reflecting the variety of different neuroendocrine cell types of the foregut area, including entero-chromaffin cells (EC), enterochromaffin-Like cells (ECL), gastrin, somatostatin, and G cells.

EARLY RECOGNITION OF A NEUROENDOCRINE CELL GENESIS

In 1926, about the same time that a consensus was being reached on the relationship between entero-chromaffin or NEC and carcinoids, a hitherto unre-ported small-cell tumor ("oat-celled sarcoma") of the mediastinum was reported by Barnard.[27] Thereafter, although Hamperl would describe the specific entity of bronchial carcinoid (1937),[30] mis-perceptions existed in the pathologic community between the precise terminology and the differ-ences or similarities between oat-cell and small-cell cancers, carcinoid tumors, and a variety of pulmonary neoplasms that exhibited components with neuroendocrine cell differentiation. Concepts relating to pulmonary NETs were notably published from the Hammersmith Hospital, London and ranged from Pearse's[24] enunciation of the APUD concept in the 1960s to Azzopardi's amplification of the histologic description in 1959,[33] wherein he identified small-cell carcinoma of the lung as a pathologic entity. Previously, the latter had been confused with a mediastinal small-cell sarcoma. Azzopardi clearly described the histology and included variants with pseudorosettes, ribbons and festoons, and spindle and insular patterns similar to the histology seen in carcinoids. He also described variation in size of the cells and DNA deposition on capillary walls, now referred to as the "Azzopardi sign." Moran and colleagues[48] in a masterly analysis of the misperceptions regarding the evolving concepts of lung NET opined that Azzopardi's descriptions themselves probably included some carcinoid tumors.

Inclusion of small-cell lung cancer with the APUD tumors was also substantiated by the work of Bensch and coworkers,[34] who described the bronchial counterpart of the Kulchitzky cells and the innervation of the bronchial glands and their relationship to peripheral carcinoid tumors, which they histologically (based on neuroendo-crine differentiation) linked to small-cell carci-noma. This proposal would subsequently be used as the basis for the development of the mod-ern concept of the pulmonary NETs. Further confirmation of the neuroendocrine relationship of these lesions was provided by reports that clearly indicated an endocrine component to the tumors. Thus, in 1956 Kincaid-Smith and Brossy[49] reported a case in which the carcinoid syndrome, due to hepatic metastases, developed 6 years af-ter lobectomy for a bronchial adenoma. Shortly thereafter, Stanford (1958) described a case of bronchial adenoma with a solitary metastasis and associated carcinoid syndrome.[50] These observa-tions were consistent with previous reports of the ill-understood association of Cushing syndrome and lung tumors that had been initially docu-mented in 1926.[51]

Skrabanek and Powell,[52] in 1978, slightly modi-fied the concept put forward by Pearse and suggested that adrenocorticotropic hormone (ACTH)–secreting tumors could be reclassified into 2 overlapping groups: the carcinoid–oat-cell group and the pheochromocytoma–neuroblastoma group. They suggested the more oat-cell-like a small-cell carcinoma appeared, the more likely it was to cause Cushing rather than carcinoid syndrome (**Fig. 10**).

THE APUD CONCEPT AND BRONCHIAL CARCINOIDS

With the evolution of more sophisticated biochem-ical techniques, the genesis of oat-cell lesions and lung carcinoids was proposed to include the ubiqui-tous polypeptide hormone–producing cells of the APUD system, which had been devised by Pearse in 1968.[53] Pearse had concluded that all such tu-mors (neural crest–related) comprised cells capable of secreting a variety of polypeptide hormones, including catecholamines and 5-hydroxytrypta-mine and possessed the common cytochemical characteristics that enabled them to be classified as part of a common neuroendocrine-based dis-ease process. It was therefore accepted that a wide variety of tumors all arising from cells of the DNES shared a commonality and could be collec-tively described as "APUDomas." The latter term, coined by the Hungarian endocrinologists Kovacs and Szijj and colleagues,[54] remained in vogue for some time before it became apparent that the orig-inal Pearse theory was flawed, and not all endocrine tumors could be co-classified. Pearse's APUD concept was built on the observations of the Aus-trian pathologist, Feyrter, who had originally recog-nized the interface of the divergent elements (neural and endocrine) and established the concept of the DNES (**Fig. 11**). His pathologic descriptions of the specialized NEC producing biologically active sub-stances and regulating homeostasis by a network functioning via endocrine, paracrine, and neura-crine mechanisms, rather than that of an "organ-based" regulation, laid the basis for contemporary understanding of gut function. Of note, Feyrter,[55] in 1938, had identified the clear cells (*Helle Zellen*) of the pancreas and gastrointestinal tract. It was

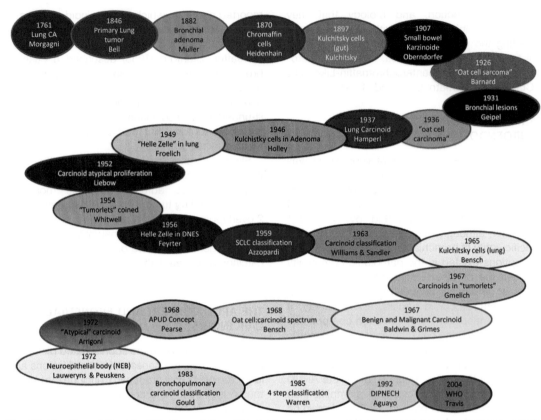

Fig. 10. Timeline of the identification of the cells and tumor types comprising bronchopulmonary neuroendocrine neoplasia. Based on the original anatomico-pathological observations by Morgagni, Bell, and Muller in the eighteenth and nineteenth century, a series of cell-based studies were developed that facilitated identification of specific tumor types. Tumor and cellular observations from the intestine (Oberndorfer and Kulchitsky) provided the basis for the documentation of the neuroendocrine origin of BPNETs, the identification of the histogenesis of neoplasia, and the delineation of benign and malignant subtypes. The latter allowed for the evolution of a series of classification systems. (*Courtesy of* Irvin M. Modlin, MD, New Haven, CT.)

this cell type that was incorporated into Pearse's APUD concept (**Fig. 12**).

THE ROLE OF IMMUNOHISTOCHEMISTRY IN THE DELINEATION OF BRONCHOPULMONARY NETS

Initial attempts to assess pulmonary NETS and define neuroendocrine differentiation were based on the use of standard hematoxylin and eosin (H&E) morphology. Introduction of staining techniques enabled a further classification into argentaffin and argyrophilic lesions. However, the subsequent development of immunohistochemical techniques greatly augmented the ability to define neuroendocrine lesions.

During the first half of the twentieth century, silver stains attained significance in the identification not only of various neural cell types but also in visualization of endocrine cells, especially those in the gastrointestinal tract. As early as 1914,

Masson described a silver method that later was found to visualize an endocrine cell population of the gastrointestinal tract.[56] Other silver stains, developed between 1930 and 1960, were able to identify a larger population of endocrine cells than the Masson stain. These stains included the Gros-Schulze silver technique and the Bodian protargol stain.[57] The latter method especially was used fairly commonly for demonstrating endocrine cells in different organs and tumors including the lung.[58] In 1960, Hellerstrom and Hellman modified a silver method developed by Davenport in 1930[59] for nervous tissue.[60] Subsequently, Sevier and Munger[61] (1965) described a silver nitrate stain for nerve structures, and 3 years later Black and Haffner[62] (1968) found that this stain also demonstrated a cell population in the human stomach and cells in a multifocal gastric carcinoid tumor.

In 1968, Grimelius described another silver stain, which in conjunction with the work of Pearse, Polak, and Bloom, led to a more

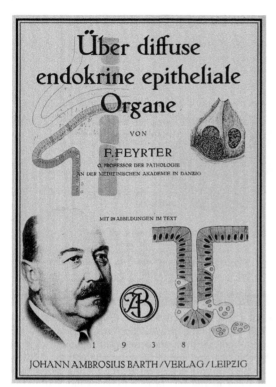

Über diffuse
endokrine epitheliale
Organe

VON

F. FEYRTER

O. PROFESSOR DER PATHOLOGIE
AN DER MEDIZINISCHEN AKADEMIE IN DANZIG

MIT 28 ABBILDUNGEN IM TEXT

1 9 3 8

JOHANN AMBROSIUS BARTH / VERLAG / LEIPZIG

Fig. 11. In 1938, Friedrich Feyrter (1895–1973), while at the Medical Academy of Danzig, published his seminal paper describing *"Helle Zellen"* (clear cells) in the ducts of the pancreas and mucous membrane of the gastrointestinal tract. This text identified and characterized the role of specialized NEC producing biologically active substances and regulating homeostasis by a network functioning via endocrine, paracrine, and neuracrine mechanisms and established the basis for his DNES classification (1956). This observation, in addition to providing the foundation for the APUD concept, allowed for the recognition of the neuroendocrine basis of BPNET. (*Courtesy of* Irvin M. Modlin, MD, New Haven, CT.)

sophisticated understanding of the neuroendocrine features of pulmonary tumors (**Fig. 13**). Gould, in 1983,[63] initially described the neuroendocrine bodies and the NEC, which undergo hyperplasia in certain types of injuries and documented their neuroendocrine products (serotonin, bombesin, calcitonin, leu-enkephalin, and somatostatin). Warren and colleagues,[64] in 1984 reported additional neuropeptides produced by pulmonary carcinoids (prolactin, vasoactive intestinal polypeptide, growth hormone-releasing hormone, chorionic gonadotropin, melanocyte-stimulating hormone, endorphin, and pancreatic polypeptide).[64] Thereafter, in 1988, Linnoila, and subsequently, Gould, described the high incidence of more general markers of NETs by demonstrating staining for chromogranin A, synaptophysin and neuron-specific enolase.[65,66]

PULMONARY NEUROENDOCRINE CELLS AND NEUROEPITHELIAL BODIES

As early as 1949, it was apparent to Froelich that clear cells, or "Helle Zelle," were present in the bronchial mucosa of man and other animals arranged singly or in corpuscular aggregates, termed, *"Knoetchen."*[67] He proposed that they were of neuroectodermal origin and might subserve a chemoreceptive function. Shortly thereafter in 1956, Feyrter[55] confirmed the existence of these cells and concluded that they represented the pulmonary component of the DNES that he had originally described in 1938. An amplification of the concept was provided in 1972 when Lauweryns and Peuskens[68] of Leuwen extended the original contributions of Froelich's bronchial clear cell aggregates in their 1969 studies of neonatal lungs and termed them neuroepithelial bodies (NEBs).

Lung tissue comprises numerous different component cell types variously related to the maintenance of gas exchange and sampling of the environment. Within this complex heterogeneous matrix, pulmonary neuroendocrine cells (PNEC) represent a group of specialized airway epithelial cells that occur as solitary cells (1/2500 epithelial cells) or as clusters referred to as NEB.[69] NEB cells exhibit mechanosensory properties and "stretch"-induced NEB cell 5-Hydroxy-Tryptamine release is mediated by mechanosensitive ion channels. Lauweryns and Preuskens, who had described NEBs in the respiratory bronchial mucosa and distinguished them from single neuroepithelial cells, considered that both exhibited APUD features and proposed that NEBs might be the sites at which NETs arose.[68]

PNECS are of endodermal origin and located throughout the entire respiratory tract from the trachea to the terminal airways resembling classical open NEC. In this respect, they are elongated and pyramidal, contain secretory granules, and exhibit apical sensory microvilli, which project into the airway lumen. On stimulation (eg, hypoxia), PNECS respond by degranulation and exocytosis of amines and neuropeptides, which exert a local paracrine and neurocrine effect on neighboring cells and activate both extrinsic and intrinsic neurons.

PNECs, despite their phenotypic similarity to neurons, are the first cell type to form and differentiate within the primitive epithelium. Thereafter, the PNEC/NEB complex represents the lung stem cell niche that is central to airway epithelial regeneration and lung carcinogenesis. Although most PNECs exist as sparsely distributed solitary cells,

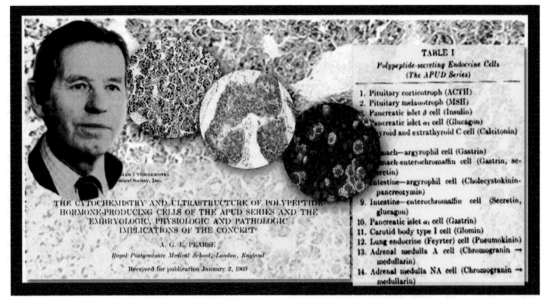

Fig. 12. Anthony Pearse (1916–2003) developed the concept of a histochemically derived APUD cell lineage (*frontispiece; bottom left*). This proposal was derived from earlier work describing "*Helle Zellen*" in different organs as well as Feyrter's anatomic description of the DNES. Pearse identified that most endocrine cells regardless of their location (lung, gut, and so on) shared a common series of biochemical and immunostaining characteristics (chromogranin A, *top left*; synaptophysin, *center*; pancreatic β-cell preparation, *center right*). His postulate of a common origin (the neural crest) for these cells, although useful, subsequently was proven to be invalid. Within this classification, Pearse considered the lung endocrine cell, the Feyrter cell, to be an APUD cell (*right bottom*) characterized by its putative product "pneumokinin." (*Courtesy of* Irvin M. Modlin, MD, New Haven, CT.)

some are aggregated in innervated PNEC clusters referred to as NEBs. Both solitary PNECs and NEBs exhibit similar phenotypes in terms of storage of a profile of bioactive amines and peptides and represent the cell source of bronchopulmonary carcinoids. The relationship of pluripotent progenitor cell populations including Clara cells is unclear. The latter were initially described as a morphologically distinct cell type by von Kolliker in 1881, but named by Clara (1899–1966) in 1937, as a consequence of his experimental studies of animal bronchioles.[70] Clara cells are considered pivotal in protecting the airway from environmental exposures based on their diverse functions in lung homeostasis, including roles in xenobiotic metabolism, immune system regulation, and progenitor cell activity. This function may well be related to the similar activity of the NEC of the gut that sample luminal nutrients or regulate blood flow, secretion, and mucosal proliferation. It is likely that either a luminal stimulus (in the case of gut NE cells) or an airway agent may play a role in the initiation of both gut and bronchial NETs.

THE CONTINUUM OF BRONCHOPULMONARY NEUROENDOCRINE TUMORS

The lesions have been identified to range from central in location to peripheral and the cells of origin variously considered as components of the DNES, APUD in origin, or specifically Kulchitsky in type. The spectrum of tumors ranges from modest hyperplasias and tumorlets via adenomas and carcinoids to atypical lesions and highly aggressive malignancies typified as carcinomas. Although many are benign or low-grade malignant neoplasms without evident cause and with few significant clinical implications, some are functional (secrete bioactive products) and others are highly aggressive with local and distant metastasis.

PERIPHERAL CARCINOIDS—A TOPOGRAPHIC CONCEPT

Gmelich and coworkers[71] described Kulchitzky-type cells proliferating in the periphery of the lung in association with multiple peripheral carcinoid tumors in 1967 and suggested that these cells were the origin of peripheral pulmonary carcinoids. Subsequently, in 1976, Bonikos, working with the same group at Yale, described 5 cases of peripheral carcinoid tumors, which they distinguished from the more usual type of bronchial carcinoid by location in distal airways.[72] In 1980, Ranchod and Levine[73] published a series of 35 cases of spindle cell peripheral carcinoid tumors of the lung. All of the patients had a single tumor with

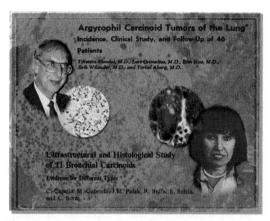

Fig. 13. Lars Grimelius (*top left*) developed a silver nitrate–based method in 1968 with fewer technical difficulties than earlier versions, which provided a reproducible stain for a range of endocrine cell types. The efficacy of this argyrophil stain was demonstrated for lung tumors in 1980; 93% of tumors stained positive with the Grimelius stain (*top*). Julia Polak (*bottom right*) at the Hammersmith with Bloom and Pearse developed a series of immunohistochemical assays based on the individual peptides produced by endocrine cells. This approach became of considerable utility in establishing the neuroendocrine specificity of lung lesions as evident in substance P staining of BPNETs (*bottom*). The combination of Grimelius' histologic technique in conjunction with the immunohistochemical approach of Polak led to a more sophisticated delineation of the neuroendocrine features of bronchopulmonary tumors. (*Courtesy of Irvin M. Modlin, MD, New Haven, CT.*)

lesions that were well circumscribed. Atypical mitotic figures, necrosis, and vascular deposition of DNA were not noted but Kulchitzky cell proliferation was evident in the surrounding lung of 5 of 13 cases. This landmark series of peripheral carcinoid tumors did not indicate a particularly aggressive behavior for them as a group but suggested an association between neuroendocrine hyperplasia, tumorlets, and peripheral carcinoids.

BRONCHIAL CARCINOIDS (TYPICAL)

Although the classical description of a bronchial carcinoid was first provided by Hamperl in 1937,[30] more recent appreciations of bronchopulmonary carcinoid (BPC) were provided by DeLellis and colleagues in 1984.[74] They noted that BPC most closely resembled the "benign" carcinoid lesions of the gut first described by Oberndorfer, who had described their characteristic insular, trabecular, or mixed pattern histologic appearance. DeLellis observed that this fundamental description still served as the basis of recognition of carcinoids in extraintestinal

locations, including the lung. Although diverse histologic criteria have been described for the recognition of neuroendocrine neoplasms, it is unusual for H&E to identify a bronchopulmonary carcinoid, which is especially true of the typical proximal BPCs, which occur in cartilage-bearing bronchi. These lesions most resemble the mature neuroendocrine components of the lung and are probably derived from mature endocrine cells or from embryonic cells committed to differentiation as NEC. DeLellis suggested that the term carcinoid be restricted to bronchopulmonary neoplasms composed of 5-hydroxytryptamine (serotonin)-producing enterochromaffin-type cells.

ATYPICAL BRONCHIAL CARCINOID

In 1972, Arrigoni and colleagues[75] from the Mayo Clinic recognized that although carcinoids generally have a good prognosis, some metastasized and a rare few progressed to systemic spread and death. They undertook a classic surgical pathology study to identify predictive histologic factors of more aggressive behavior in 215 carcinoid tumors of the lung. In 23 carcinoid tumors, they identified a series of features that allowed them to describe the entity of the atypical carcinoid. These features included an increased number of mitotic figures, pleomorphism or irregularity of the nuclei with prominent nucleoli hyperchromatism and an abnormal (increased) nuclear-cytoplasmic ratio, areas of increased cellularity with disorganization of the architecture, and areas of tumor necrosis. Arrigoni and colleagues concluded that two-thirds of atypical carcinoids occur in men, that the group comprises ~10% of bronchial carcinoids, and overall exhibits a worse prognosis than the typical ones. Ten years later, Mills and coworkers[76] described a group of atypical carcinoids, which more closely resembled small-cell lung cancer; areas of small-cell lung cancer were found in 5 of their 17 cases.

PULMONARY NEUROENDOCRINE HYPERPLASIA

The recognition of the entity of diffuse idiopathic pulmonary neuroendocrine cell hyperplasia (DIPNECH) was initially described by Aguayo and colleagues in 1992.[77] It is now considered to be a precursor lesion that culminates in the development of BPCs. The cause of pulmonary neuroendocrine hyperplasia is unclear but environmental stress (eg, high altitudes) and injuries (eg, chronic cough or obstruction) are associated with the proliferation of both PNECs and NEBs. The consequences of such events culminate in a generalized proliferation of PNECs and NEBs or a linear proliferation of PNECs and culminate in the preneoplastic condition known as DIPNECH.

Armas and coworkers,[78] in 1995, were the first to describe a case of diffuse pulmonary endocrine cell hyperplasia in which there was a florid proliferation of neuroendocrine-appearing cells proliferating on the surface of the airways and forming nodules in the alveolar spaces. Because these cells were focally positive for neuron-specific enolase with focal argyrophilia but negative for the other neuroendocrine markers, including chromogranin, serotonin, calcitonin, bombesin, and ACTH, it was suggested that this condition represented the borderline between hyperplasia and neoplasia of PNEC.

When PNECs extend beyond the basement membrane, the proliferation has been termed a "tumorlet," which can be further defined as being localized or diffuse. Thus, a nodular PNEC proliferation of NEC that constitutes a nodule less than 5 mm in size was referred to as a pulmonary carcinoid tumorlet. Proliferations comprising nodules greater than 5 mm in diameter thereafter became classified as carcinoid tumors. DIPNECH is considered to represent a preinvasive lesion for carcinoid tumors. Neuroendocrine cell hyperplasia and tumorlets are also associated with inflammation and fibrosis (a reactive response) and may also be identified in lung in up to 75% of carcinoid tumors.

CHEMODECTOMA (PARAGANGLIOMA)

In 1958, Heppleston described a carotid-body-like tumor of the lung in a Welsh coal worker who was found by screening chest radiograph to have a small rounded opacity that slightly increased in size over 6 years.[79] This opacity was demonstrated to be a paraganglioma-like carcinoid. The distinction of carcinoids, especially from the periphery of the lung, from paragangliomas and chemodectomas is of historical interest and continuing debate. Most peripheral tumors with the histologic appearance of a typical carcinoid tumor or with a spindle-cell pattern and neuroendocrine markers have been considered carcinoids. In 1990, Barbareschi and coworkers[80] published an immunohistochemical study of 46 typical bronchial carcinoids that identified that in 18 of them (39%), a biphasic pattern consistent with paragangliomatous insular cell groups surrounded by abundant stellate S-100 protein-positive sustenacular cells was evident. They described these biphasic carcinoids as "paranglioid" bronchial carcinoids and noted that gastrointestinal carcinoids, pheochromocytomas, and paragangliomas also contained stellate-shaped cells at the periphery of the balls of cells in a paragangliomatous pattern.[80] The authors interpreted the immunohistochemical findings as showing Schwannian or sustenacular differentiation indicating that some of the bronchial carcinoids are more like paragangliomas.

LARGE-CELL NEUROENDOCRINE CARCINOMA

In 1985, Hammond and Sause[81] described a group of 8 histologically large-cell undifferentiated carcinomas, which were shown to have neuroendocrine differentiation by immunohistochemistry. They were compared with 9 bronchial carcinoids and 9 atypical carcinoids. All of the typical carcinoids were recognized by light microscopy, and all of these patients were alive and free of disease at the end of the follow-up period.

CARCINOID, WELL-DIFFERENTIATED NEUROENDOCRINE CARCINOMA, INTERMEDIATE NEUROENDOCRINE CARCINOMA, AND SMALL-CELL NEUROENDOCRINE CARCINOMA

In 1985, Warren and coworkers[82] proposed a 4-step classification of the neuroendocrine carcinomas: typical carcinoids, well-differentiated neuroendocrine carcinomas, intermediate neuroendocrine carcinomas, and small-cell neuroendocrine carcinomas. The typical carcinoids were usually centrally placed, displayed little or no pleomorphism, were richly granulated by electron microscopy, and were strongly positive by immunohistochemistry. The hormones they displayed were indigenous to their site of origin: serotonin, bombesin, and calcitonin. Metastases were rare. Well-differentiated carcinomas were the so-called atypical carcinoids as well as cases misinterpreted as early oat-cell carcinoma.

THE CLASSIFICATION CONUNDRUM

As the delineation of bronchopulmonary NETs moved from descriptive pathologic abnormality to morphologic detail and then embraced histochemistry, a variety of progressive perceptions of the nature of neuroendocrine lung neoplasms emerged over time. The steady addition of information predictably therefore has led to the development several classification systems. Although logical in their individual construct, there remains a need to establish a definitive system to categorize this complex group of tumors.

In 1977, Gould[83] adapted the current vogue of using the concept of the APUD system to explain tumor relationships by introducing the terms neuroendocrinomas and neuroendocrine carcinomas to describe BPNs. He further advocated that traditional terms such as bronchial adenoma should be discarded because they did not convey the true nature of these neoplasms and inferred that "oat-cell" carcinomas represent the malignant counterpart of carcinoid.

In 1983, Gould[63] proposed a new classification system for neuroendocrine pulmonary neoplasms seeking to better define the term carcinoid based on the consideration that the term had been overused and provoked unnecessary confusion. This new classification system emphasized the unclear distinction between some carcinoids termed pleomorphic, atypical, and anaplastic that exhibited atypical histologic features and aggressive behavior. Although this classification also sought to remove terminology, such as small-cell bronchogenic carcinoma, undifferentiated small-cell carcinoma, and anaplastic small-cell carcinoma, this area remained ambiguous. Nevertheless, the Gould classification system was useful in

recognizing 4 categories of BPNETs: bronchopulmonary carcinoid, well-differentiated neuroendocrine carcinoma, neuroendocrine carcinoma of intermediate-sized cells, and neuroendocrine carcinoma of small cell type.

In 1985, Paladugu and colleagues,[84] reverting to the archaic terminology of NEC, presented an alternative classification system wherein they considered such lesions to be bronchopulmonary Kulchitsky cell carcinomas (KCCs).[84] This system classified neuroendocrine neoplasms into 3 types, namely, KCC-I, KCC-II, and KCC-III for typical carcinoid, atypical carcinoid, and small-cell carcinoma, respectively.

In 1995, Capella and coworkers[85] once again revised the classification of NET of the lung, pancreas, and gut into 3 groups: (1) benign or low-grade malignant, non-functioning, well-differentiated tumor as the equivalent for conventional carcinoid; (2) low-grade malignant, nonfunctioning, well-differentiated carcinoma as equivalent for atypical carcinoid; and (3) high-grade

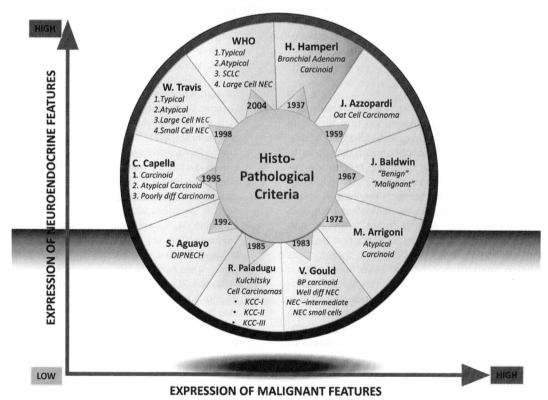

Fig. 14. Evolution of the classification of bronchopulmonary neuroendocrine neoplasia. In 1937, Herwig Hamperl provided the initial classic description of a bronchial carcinoid. Thereafter, it was noted that that oat-cell carcinomas exhibited neuroendocrine (*carcinoid*) features and as such tumors might be either benign or malignant. Defining the precise level of malignancy led to the development of a variety of classifications in the 1980s and 1990s. The subsequent recognition by Aguayo of the complexities of histogenesis and the relationship of neoplastic precursor lesions further emphasized the complexity of the spectrum of tumors constituting BPNETs. The 4-stage classification of Travis was adopted by the WHO in 2004. (*Courtesy of* Irvin M. Modlin, MD, New Haven, CT.)

malignant, functioning or nonfunctioning, poorly differentiated carcinoma for the large cell, small cell, or intermediate type.

After an initial assessment in 1991 of large-cell NET, Travis and colleagues,[86] in 1998, sought to further amplify and clarify the field by providing further definition of the 4 pulmonary neuroendocrine tumor groups and redefining the criteria for the diagnosis of carcinoid and atypical carcinoid.[87] This system transferred large-cell neuroendocrine carcinoma into the high-grade category of tumors, in contrast with his previous study.[86]

In 2002, Huang and coworkers[88] sought to amplify the Travis classification by dividing BPNETs into 5 categories. Thus, carcinoid and atypical carcinoid were separated into well-modified and moderately differentiated neuroendocrine carcinomas. Large-cell neuroendocrine carcinoma and small-cell carcinoma were retained using the modifier "undifferentiated" and an additional group, "poorly differentiated neuroendocrine carcinoma," was added. The definitive classification of BPNETs by the World Health Organization (WHO) group in 2004 provided a balanced schema allowing for a global uniform assessment of the pathologic evaluation of neuroendocrine lung tumors (**Fig. 14**).[89]

SUMMARY

In the three-quarters of a century that have elapsed since the first description of a bronchial carcinoid, the field has progressed from serendipitous radiological or bronchoscopic diagnosis to computed tomography, magnetic resonance imaging, and somatostatin receptor imaging identification. Similarly, pathologic techniques have advanced from a naïve assessment of neoplasia to a delineation of several tumor subtypes and an understanding of the neuroendocrine basis of the disease process. Endoscopic therapy has evolved from bronchoscopic resection to laser ablation and surgical ablation from sleeve resection to lobectomy and lymph node clearance. The recent usage of somatostatin receptor targeted Lutetium-177 or Yttrium-90 peptide receptor radiotherapy to treat residual disease or metastases represents the full turn of the circle as radiation, which initiated diagnosis at the turn of the nineteenth century, has now, a century later, become the novel therapeutic strategy.

Nevertheless, current pathologic analyses are limited in their ability to precisely define the malignancy of a lesion and predict the likelihood of recurrence. Diagnosis is often overlooked, detection late, and precise identification of the degree of malignancy imprecise. Similarly, therapy is largely empiric and limited in its efficacy given the inability to precisely characterize the molecular targets of a particular tumor and the paucity of specific agents.

Therefore, the issues of the future that remain to be resolved are early detection of tumors by molecular blood biomarkers, establishment of the individual genomic tumor patterns that define the biologic behavior of each tumor, and the identification of the tumor interactome and master regulators that will facilitate precisely targeted therapy. A key unresolved question is the identification of the genetic and environmental activators that are responsible for the initiation of pulmonary neuroendocrine cell proliferation and neoplastic transformation. As Laennec so long ago first learned to listen to the sound of the breathing to understand lung disease, we should now embrace the subtle susurrations of the molecular rhythms of the pulmonary neuroendocrine cell and thereby divine the secrets of its propagation and the keys of its existence.

REFERENCES

1. Morgagni G. De sedibus et causis morborum per anatomen indagatis libri quinque. Venetiis: Thypographia Remondiniana, 1761.
2. Andral G. Recherches sur l'expectoration dans les différentes maladies de poitrine. Paris: Paris; 1821.
3. Laennec R. Traite de l'auscultation mediate et des maladies des poumons et du coeur. Paris: Meriadec Laennec; 1831.
4. Adler I. Primary malignant growths of the lungs and bronchi. London: Longmans, Green and Co; 1912.
5. Harting FH, Hesse W. Lung cancer, the disease of miners in the Schneeberg mines. Vjschr gericht Med off Sank 1879;30:296–309.
6. Rottmann H. Über Primäre Lungencarcinome. Wurzberg (Germany): University of Wurzberg; 1898.
7. Williams FH. The roentgen rays in thoracic diseases. Trans Assoc Am Physicians 1897;12:314.
8. McMahon FD, Carman RD. The roentgenologic diagnosis of primary carcinoma of the lung. Am J Med Sci 1918;clv:34.
9. Jackson C. The bronchial tree: its study by insufflation of opaque substances in the living. Am J Roent 1918;5:454–5.
10. Sicard JA, Forestier J. The radiologic examination of the bronchopulmonary cavities by means of intra-tracheal injections of iodized oil. J Med Franc 1924;13:3–9.
11. Martin HE, Ellis EB. Biopsy by needle puncture and aspiration. Ann Surg 1930;22:169–81.
12. Kerley P. Neoplasms of the lungs and bronchi. Br J Radiol 1925;68:333–49.
13. Peterson HO. Benign adenoma of the bronchus. J Roentgenology 1936;36:836.

14. Allen IV. Bronchial adenoma. Can Med Assoc J 1946;55:498–501.
15. Zellos S. Bronchial adenoma. Thorax 1962;17:61–8.
16. Hattori S, Matsuda M, Sugiyama T, et al. Cytologic diagnosis of early lung cancer: brushing method under X-ray television fluoroscopy. Dis Chest 1964;45:129–42.
17. Dahlgren S. Needle biopsy of intrapulmonary hamartoma. Scand J Respir Dis 1966;47:187–94.
18. Killian G. Ueber directe Bronchoskopie. MMW 1898;27:844–7.
19. Jackson C. The bronchoscope as an aid in general diagnosis. Tr Am Laryngol Assoc NY 1914;xxxvi: 51–63.
20. Hopkins HH, Kapany NS. A flexible fibrescope, using static scanning. Nature 1954;173:39–41.
21. Becker HD, Marsh BR. History of the rigid bronchoscope. Basel (Switzerland): S. Karger; 2000.
22. Davies HM. Recent advances in the surgery of the lung and pleura. Br J Surg 1913;1:228–58.
23. Grimelius L. A silver nitrate stain for alpha-2 cells in human pancreatic islets. Acta Soc Med Ups 1968; 73:243–70.
24. Pearse AG. The cytochemistry and ultrastructure of polypeptide hormone-producing cells of the APUD series and the embryologic, physiologic and pathologic implications of the concept. J Histochem Cytochem 1969;17:303–13.
25. Polak JM, Coulling I, Bloom S, et al. Immunofluorescent localization of secretin and enteroglucagon in human intestinal mucosa. Scand J Gastroenterol 1971;6:739–44.
26. Carter D. The neuroendocrine tumors of the lung, 1926-1998: some historical observations. Semin Diagn Pathol 2008;25:154–65.
27. Barnard W. The nature of the 'oat-celled sarcoma' of the mediastinum. J Pathol 1926;29:41–4.
28. McKeown F. Oat-cell carcinoma of the oesophagus. J Pathol Bacteriol 1952;64:889–91.
29. Geipel P. Concerning our knowledge of benign bronchial tumors. Frankf Z Pathol 1931;42:516.
30. Hamperl H. Ueber gutartige Bronchialtumoren (Cylindrome und Carcinoide). Virchow's Arch (Pathol Anat) 1937;300:46.
31. Modlin IM, Shapiro MD, Kidd M. Siegfried Oberndorfer: origins and perspectives of carcinoid tumors. Hum Pathol 2004;35:1440–51.
32. Oberndorfer S. Karzinoide Tumoren des Dünndarmes. Frankf Z Pathol 1907;1:426–9.
33. Azzopardi JG. Oat-cell carcinoma of the bronchus. J Pathol Bacteriol 1959;78:513–9.
34. Bensch KG, Corrin B, Pariente R, et al. Oat-cell carcinoma of the lung. Its origin and relationship to bronchial carcinoid. Cancer 1968;22:1163–72.
35. Muller HL. Zur Entstehungsgeschichte der Bronchialerweiter ungen (inaugural dissertation). Halle (Germany): Halle University; 1882.
36. Heine J. Ueber eine primare gestielte Bronchialgeschwulst. Verh Dtsch Ges Pathol 1927;22:293.
37. Kramer R. Adenoma of bronchus. Ann Otol Rhinol Genol 1960;83.
38. Holley SW. Bronchial adenomas. Mil Surg 1946;99: 528–54.
39. Feyrter F. Ueber das Bronchuscarcinoid. Virchow's Arch (Pathol Anat) 1959;332:25–43.
40. Williams ED, Azzopardi JG. Tumours of the lung and the carcinoid syndrome. Thorax 1960;15:30–6.
41. Williams ED, Sandler M. The classification of carcinoid tum ours. Lancet 1963;1:238–9.
42. Liebow A. Tumors of the lower respiratory tract. Atlas of Tumor. Pathology (section 5, fascicle 17). Washingon, DC: Armed Forces Institute of Pathology; 1952.
43. Goodner JT, Berg JW, Watson WL. The nonbenign nature of bronchial carcinoids and cylindromas. Cancer 1961;14:539–46.
44. Weiss L, Ingram M. Adenomatoid bronchial tumors. A consideration of the carcinoid tumors and the salivary tumors of the bronchial tree. Cancer 1961;14:161–78.
45. Modlin IM, Shapiro MD, Kidd M, et al. Siegfried oberndorfer and the evolution of carcinoid disease. Arch Surg 2007;142:187–97.
46. Biorck G, Axen O, Thorson A. Unusual cyanosis in a boy with congenital pulmonary stenosis and tricuspid insufficiency. Fatal outcome after angiocardiography. Am Heart J 1952;44:143–8.
47. Moertel CG, Sauer WG, Dockerty MB, et al. Life history of the carcinoid tumor of the small intestine. Cancer 1961;14:901–12.
48. Moran CA, Suster S, Coppola D, et al. Neuroendocrine carcinomas of the lung: a critical analysis. Am J Clin Pathol 2009;131:206–21. http://dx.doi.org/10.1309/AJCP9H1OTMUCSKQW.
49. Kincaid-Smith P, Brossy JJ. A case of bronchial adenoma with liver metastasis. Thorax 1956;11: 36–40.
50. Stanford WR, Davis JE, Gunter JU, et al. Bronchial adenoma (carcinoid type) with solitary metastasis and associated functioning carcinoid syndrome. South Med J 1958;51:449–54.
51. Brown WH. A case of pluriglandular syndrome: "diabetes of bearded women". Lancet 1928;212: 1022–3.
52. Skrabanek P, Powell D. Unifying concept of nonpituitary ACTH-secreting tumors: evidence of common origin of neural-crest tumors, carcinoids, and oat-cell carcinomas. Cancer 1978;42:1263–9.
53. Carvalheira AF, Welsch U, Pearse AG. Cytochemical and ultrastructural observations on the argentaffin and argyrophil cells of the gastro-intestinal tract in mammals, and their place in the APUD series of polypeptide-secreting cells. Histochemie 1968;14:33–46.

54. Szijj I, Csapo Z, Laszlo FA, et al. Medullary cancer of the thyroid gland associated with hypercorticism. Cancer 1969;24:167–73.

55. Feyrter F. Über diffuse endokrine epitheliale Organe. Leipzig (Germany): Barth; 1938.

56. Masson P. La glande endocrine de l'intestin chez l'homme. CR Acad Sci 1914;158:59–61.

57. Bodian D. A new method for staining nerve fibres and nerve endings in mounted paraffin sections. Anat Rec 1936;65:89–97.

58. Grimelius L. A modified silver proteinate method for studying the argyrophil cells of the islet of Langerhans. In: Brolin SE, Hellman B, Knutson H, editors. The structure and metabolism of the pancreatic islets. Oxford (United Kingdom): Pergamon Press; 1964. p. 99–104.

59. Davenport HA. Staining nerve fibers in mounted sections with alcoholic silver nitrate solution. Arch Neurol Psykiat 1930;24:690–5.

60. Hellerstrom C, Hellman B. Some aspects of silver impregnation of the islets of Langerhans in the rat. Acta Endocrinol (Copenh) 1960;35:518–32.

61. Sevier AC, Munger BL. Technical note: a silver method for paraffin sections of neural tissue. J Neuropathol Exp Neurol 1965;24:130–5.

62. Black WC, Haffner HE. Diffuse hyperplasia of gastric argyrophil cells and multiple carcinoid tumors. An historical and ultrastructural study. Cancer 1968;21:1080–99.

63. Gould VE, Linnoila RI, Memoli VA, et al. Neuroendocrine components of the bronchopulmonary tract: hyperplasias, dysplasias, and neoplasms. Lab Invest 1983;49:519–37.

64. Warren WH, Memoli VA, Gould VE. Immunohistochemical and ultrastructural analysis of bronchopulmonary neuroendocrine neoplasms. I. Carcinoids. Ultrastruct Pathol 1984;6:15–27.

65. Linnoila RI, Mulshine JL, Steinberg SM, et al. Neuroendocrine differentiation in endocrine and nonendocrine lung carcinomas. Am J Clin Pathol 1988;90:641–52.

66. Gould VE, Lee I, Warren WH. Immunohistochemical evaluation of neuroendocrine cells and neoplasms of the lung. Pathol Res Pract 1988;183:200–13.

67. Froelich F. Die helle Zelle der Bronchialschleimhaut und ihre Beziehungen zum Problem der Chemoreceptoren. Frankf Z Pathol 1949;60:517–59.

68. Lauweryns JM, Peuskens JC. Neuro-epithelial bodies (neuroreceptor or secretory organs?) in human infant bronchial and bronchiolar epithelium. Anat Rec 1972;172:471–81.

69. Gustafsson BI, Kidd M, Chan A, et al. Bronchopulmonary neuroendocrine tumors. Cancer 2008;113:5–21.

70. Clara M. Zur Histobiologie des Bronchalepithels. Z Mikrosk Anat Forsch 1937;41:321–47.

71. Gmelich JT, Bensch KG, Liebow AA. Cells of Kultschitzky type in bronchioles and their relation to the origin of peripheral carcinoid tumor. Lab Invest 1967;17:88–98.

72. Bonikos DS, Bensch KG, Jamplis RW. Peripheral pulmonary carcinoid tumors. Cancer 1976;37:1977–98.

73. Ranchod M, Levine GD. Spindle-cell carcinoid tumors of the lung: a clinicopathologic study of 35 cases. Am J Surg Pathol 1980;4:315–31.

74. DeLellis RA, Dayal Y, Wolfe HJ. Carcinoid tumors. Changing concepts and new perspectives. Am J Surg Pathol 1984;8:295–300.

75. Arrigoni MG, Woolner LB, Bernatz PE. Atypical carcinoid tumors of the lung. J Thorac Cardiovasc Surg 1972;64:413–21.

76. Mills SE, Cooper PH, Walker AN, et al. Atypical carcinoid tumor of the lung. A clinicopathologic study of 17 cases. Am J Surg Pathol 1982;6:643–54.

77. Aguayo SM, Miller YE, Waldron JA Jr, et al. Brief report: idiopathic diffuse hyperplasia of pulmonary neuroendocrine cells and airways disease. N Engl J Med 1992;327:1285–8.

78. Armas OA, White DA, Erlandson RA, et al. Diffuse idiopathic pulmonary neuroendocrine cell proliferation presenting as interstitial lung disease. Am J Surg Pathol 1995;19:963–70.

79. Heppleston AG. A carotid-body-like tumour in the lung. J Pathol Bacteriol 1958;75:461–4.

80. Barbareschi M, Frigo B, Mosca L, et al. Bronchial carcinoids with S-100 positive sustentacular cells. A comparative study with gastrointestinal carcinoids, pheochromocytomas and paragangliomas. Pathol Res Pract 1990;186:212–22.

81. Hammond ME, Sause WT. Large cell neuroendocrine tumors of the lung. Clinical significance and histopathologic definition. Cancer 1985;56:1624–9.

82. Warren WH, Gould VE, Faber LP, et al. Neuroendocrine neoplasms of the bronchopulmonary tract. A classification of the spectrum of carcinoid to small cell carcinoma and intervening variants. J Thorac Cardiovasc Surg 1985;89:819–25.

83. Gould VE. Neuroendocrinomas and neuroendocrine carcinomas: APUD cell system neoplasms and their aberrant secretory activities. Pathol Annu 1977;12:33–62.

84. Paladugu RR, Benfield JR, Pak HY, et al. Bronchopulmonary Kulchitzky cell carcinomas. A new classification scheme for typical and atypical carcinoids. Cancer 1985;55:1303–11.

85. Capella C, Heitz PU, Hofler H, et al. Revised classification of neuroendocrine tumours of the lung, pancreas and gut. Virchows Arch 1995;425:547–60.

86. Travis WD, Linnoila RI, Tsokos MG, et al. Neuroendocrine tumors of the lung with proposed criteria for large-cell neuroendocrine carcinoma. An

ultrastructural, immunohistochemical, and flow cytometric study of 35 cases. Am J Surg Pathol 1991;15:529–53.

87. Travis WD, Gal AA, Colby TV, et al. Reproducibility of neuroendocrine lung tumor classification. Hum Pathol 1998;29:272–9.

88. Huang Q, Muzitansky A, Mark EJ. Pulmonary neuroendocrine carcinomas. A review of 234 cases and a statistical analysis of 50 cases treated at one institution using a simple clinicopathologic classification. Arch Pathol Lab Med 2002;126:545–53.

89. Travis WD, Brambilla E, Muller-Hermlink H, et al. World Health Organization classification of tumours. Pathology and genetics of tumours of the lung, pleura, thymus and heart. Lyon (France): IARC Press; 2004.

90. Graham EA, Singer JJ. Successful removal of an entire lung for carcinoma of bronchus. JAMA 1933;101:1011371–4.

91. Gloyme SR. A case of oat-cell carcinoma of the lung occurring in asbestosis. Tubercule 1936;18: 100–1.

92. Eloesser L. Transthoracic bronchotomy for removal of benign tumors of the bronchus. Ann Surg 1940; 112:1067–70.

93. Prior JT. Minute peripheral pulmonary tumors; observations on their histogenesis. Am J Pathol 1953;29:703–19.

94. Felton WL 2nd, Liebow AA, Lindskog GE. Peripheral and multiple bronchial adenomas. Cancer 1953;6:555–67.

95. Whitwell L. Tumourlets of the lung. J Pathol Bacteriol 1955;70:529–41.

96. Price-Thomas C. Surgical treatment of lung cancer. Brux Med 1955;35:2065–75 [in French].

97. Bensch KG, Gordon GB, Miller LR. Electron microscopic and biochemical studies on the bronchial carcinoid tumor. Cancer 1965;18:592–602.

98. Baldwin JN, Grimes OF. Bronchial adenomas. Surg Gynecol Obstet 1967;124:813–8.

99. Bergsagel DE, Jenkin RD, Pringle JF, et al. Lung cancer: clinical trial of radiotherapy alone vs. radiotherapy plus cyclophosphamide. Cancer 1972;30: 621–7.

100. Churg A, Warnock ML. Pulmonary tumorlet. A form of peripheral carcinoid. Cancer 1976;37:1469–77.

101. Godwin JD 2nd, Brown CC. Comparative epidemiology of carcinoid and oat-cell tumors of the lung. Cancer 1977;40:1671–3.

102. Ranchod M. The histogenesis and development of pulmonary tumorlets. Cancer 1977;39:1135–45.

103. Gould VE, Linnoila RI, Memoli VA, et al. Neuroendocrine cells and neuroendocrine neoplasms of the lung. Pathol Annu 1983;18:287–330.

104. Maini CL, Tofani A, Venturo I, et al. Somatostatin receptor imaging in small cell lung cancer using 111In-DTPA-octreotide: a preliminary study. Nucl Med Commun 1993;14:962–8.

105. Iser G, Pfohl M, Dorr U, et al. Ectopic ACTH secretion due to a bronchopulmonary carcinoid localized by somatostatin receptor scintigraphy. Clin Investig 1994;72:887–91.

Pathology and Diagnosis of Neuroendocrine Tumors: Lung Neuroendocrine

William D. Travis, MD

KEYWORDS

- Carcinoid • Typical carcinoid • Atypical carcinoid • Large cell neuroendocrine carcinoma
- Small cell carcinoma • Neuroendocrine • Lung • Neuroendocrine cell hyperplasia

KEY POINTS

- Neuroendocrine tumors of the lung represent a spectrum of low-grade typical carcinoid (TC), intermediate-grade atypical carcinoid (AC), and high-grade large cell neuroendocrine carcinoma (LCNEC) and small cell lung carcinoma (SCLC).
- The most important histologic feature used to distinguish the grade of lung NE tumors is the mitotic count.
- Unlike in the gastrointestinal tract, Ki-67 is not established as a way to distinguish TC from AC. However, it is very useful for the separation of carcinoid tumors from the high-grade LCNEC and SCLC, particularly in small biopsies with crush artifact.

INTRODUCTION: NATURE OF THE PROBLEM

Neuroendocrine (NE) tumors of the lung range from the low-grade typical carcinoid (TC) and intermediate-grade atypical carcinoid (AC) to the high-grade large cell neuroendocrine carcinoma (LCNEC) and small cell lung carcinoma (SCLC) (**Box 1**).[1,2] SCLC is the most common NE lung tumor, representing approximately 14% of invasive lung cancers.[3] LCNEC represents about 3% of lung cancers in surgical series. Carcinoid tumors account for 1% to 2% of invasive lung malignancies. AC are the rarest of the lung NE tumors. Comprising approximately 10% of all carcinoids, they account for only about 0.1% to 0.2% of lung cancers.[4] Diffuse idiopathic neuroendocrine cell hyperplasia (DIPNECH) is a very rare condition, characterized by widespread tumorlets and NE cell hyperplasia, which represents a preinvasive lesion for carcinoid tumors (**Fig. 1**). The pathologic diagnosis of TC and SCLC is straightforward in most cases, and can be made based on light microscopy. However, it is difficult to diagnose AC and LCNEC in small biopsies or cytology, and a definitive diagnosis usually requires a surgical specimen. Therapy for TC and SCLC is primarily surgery and chemotherapy, respectively. However, the best therapy for AC and LCNEC is not established.[4]

In this article, basic principles of diagnostic pathology of pulmonary NE tumors are presented, with emphasis on the pathology, diagnostic criteria (**Box 2**), and their implications for treatment.

RELEVANT ANATOMY AND PATHOPHYSIOLOGY
Molecular Changes in Pulmonary Neuroendocrine Tumors

Recent molecular studies by the Clinical Lung Cancer Genome Project (CLCGP) clearly show that carcinoids show relatively few genetic changes when compared with the high-grade SCLC and LCNEC, supporting the concept in the 2004 World Health Organization (WHO)

Department of Pathology, Memorial Sloan Kettering Cancer Center, 1275 York Avenue, New York, NY 10021, USA
E-mail address: travisw@mskcc.org

Thorac Surg Clin 24 (2014) 257–266
http://dx.doi.org/10.1016/j.thorsurg.2014.04.001

classification that these are 2 very different groups of tumors.[5] Both SCLC and LCNEC frequently show mutations in TP53, RB1, and EP300. Additional genetic changes, such as copy number, can be found in some LCNEC that are characteristic of adenocarcinoma or squamous cell carcinoma,[5] which is compatible with the known existence of combined LCNEC where components of these other histologies are also present.

Fernandez-Cuesta and colleagues[6] recently showed that carcinoid tumors show frequent mutations in chromatin remodeling genes. Mutations were found in covalent histone modifiers in 40%

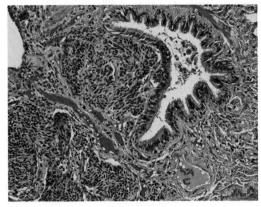

Fig. 1. Diffuse idiopathic neuroendocrine cell hyperplasia (DIPNECH). This tumorlet from a patient with DIPNECH consists of nodular clusters of neuroendocrine cells in a peribronchiolar location, causing compression of the bronchiolar lumen (Hematoxylin and eosin ×20).

and in subunits of the *SWI/SNF* complex in 22.2% of cases, with *MEN1, PSIP1,* and *ARID1A* often being affected.

Onuki and colleagues[7] analyzed pulmonary NE tumors for loss of heterozygosity (LOH) for 3p, RB, 5q21, 9p, and p53. LOH was found more often in the high-grade LCNEC and SCLC than in the carcinoids. 5q21 LOH was significantly more frequent in SCLC than in LCNEC. p53 analyzed by 3 modalities, namely immunohistochemistry, LOH, and mutation analysis, showed an increasing frequency of changes from TC to AC and the high-grade SCLC and LCNEC.[7] p53 mutations were absent in TC but present in 25% of AC, 59% of LCNEC, and 71% of SCLC. These results are supported by other studies showing that high-grade NE carcinomas have p53 expression ranging between 40% and 86%, and p53 mutations ranging from 27% to 59%.[8–10]

DIAGNOSIS
Small Cell Carcinoma

Clinical features

SCLC is the most common pulmonary NE tumor, with more than 30,000 cases anticipated to be diagnosed in the United States in 2014.[11] There has been a decrease in the frequency of SCLC cases over the past 30 years in the United States from 17% to 13% of all lung cancers, according to the United States National Cancer Institute Surveillance, Epidemiologic, and End Results (SEER) database.[3,12] Most patients present with advanced disease, but in approximately 5% of cases tumors can present as a solitary lung nodule, the latter being those that are often surgically resected.

Pathology

The diagnosis of SCLC is primarily based on light microscopy (**Fig. 2**). Tumor cells grow in sheets and nests with frequent necrosis that is often extensive. Most tumors show necrosis that may be extensive. Tumor cells are round to fusiform, typically have scant cytoplasm, and measure less than the diameter of 3 small resting lymphocytes, with finely granular nuclear chromatin. Nucleoli are inconspicuous or absent.[2,13] There is a high mitotic rate, averaging 60 to 80 per 2 mm². In some small biopsies, mitoses can difficult to identify. SCLC can readily be diagnosed in small specimens such as bronchoscopic biopsies, fine-needle aspirates, core biopsies, and

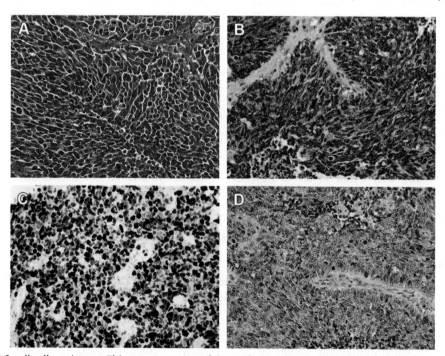

Fig. 2. (*A*) Small cell carcinoma. This tumor consists of dense sheets of small cells with scant cytoplasm and finely granular nuclear chromatin; frequent mitoses and nucleoli are inconspicuous or absent (Hematoxylin and eosin ×40). (*B*) Chromogranin is positive with a cytoplasmic granular pattern in this small cell lung carcinoma (SCLC) (Chromogranin immunohistochemistry ×40). (*C*) Ki-67 shows a high proliferation rate with almost 100% staining of tumor cells (Ki-67 immunohistochemistry ×40). (*D*) This surgically resected SCLC shows somewhat larger tumor cells that are sometimes confused with large cell neuroendocrine carcinoma (LCNEC). However, the cytologic features fit SCLC best (Hematoxylin and eosin ×40).

cytology. This identification is necessary because of the presentation in advanced stages for most patients.

There has been considerable evolution in the subtyping of SCLC, dating back to 1962 when Kreyberg[14] proposed the oat cell and polygonal subtypes (**Table 1**). Three subtypes of SCLC were proposed in the 1981 WHO classification: (1) oat cell carcinoma, (2) intermediate cell type, and (3) combined oat cell carcinoma.[15] The International Association for the Study of Lung Cancer (IASLC) proposed in 1988 to drop the category of intermediate cell type, because this could not be reproduced by expert lung cancer pathologists and significant survival differences were not demonstrable. A new category of mixed small cell/large cell carcinoma subtype was proposed, with the impression that these patients had a worse prognosis than other SCLC patients.[16] Combined SCLC was proposed for SCLC that had a component of adenocarcinoma or squamous cell carcinoma.[16] In the 1999 WHO classification the category of mixed small cell/large cell carcinoma was dropped, owing to difficulties with reproducibility for this subtype and data indicating that the prognosis was not always worse than for other SCLC.[17,18] Only 2 subtypes of SCLC were proposed in the 2004 WHO classification: SCLC with pure SCLC histology, and combined SCLC (with a mixture of any non–small cell type) (see **Boxes 1** and **2**).[2]

Combined SCLC is diagnosed when SCLC also has a component of non-SCLC (NSCLC) such as adenocarcinoma, squamous cell carcinoma, large cell carcinoma, spindle cell carcinoma, and giant cell carcinoma. Each non–small cell component present should be mentioned in the diagnosis of these tumors.[2,13] In surgically resected cases, combined SCLC may occur in up to 28% of cases.[2,13] At least 10% large or giant cells should be present for the diagnosis of combined SCLC and large cell carcinoma, but for the components of adenocarcinoma, squamous cell carcinoma, or spindle cell carcinoma the amount does not matter.[2,13]

SCLC must be separated from NSCLC (such as adenocarcinoma, large cell carcinoma, and basaloid squamous cell carcinoma), other NE lung tumors (including carcinoids and LCNEC), chronic inflammation, malignant lymphoma, malignant melanoma, and metastatic carcinomas. The most important special stain is a good-quality hematoxylin and eosin (H&E) stain.[19] Problems in the diagnosis often result from sections that are too thick or poorly stained. These problems can often be resolved by asking for recut sections from the block to make a good-quality H&E-stained section. If the histologic features are classic the diagnosis can be established by H&E alone, and immunohistochemistry may not be needed. The criteria for distinguishing SCLC from NSCLC are summarized in **Table 2**. This separation should not rest on a single feature such as cell size or nucleoli, but incorporation of multiple additional features including nuclear to cytoplasmic ratio, nuclear chromatin, nucleoli, nuclear molding, cell shape (fusiform vs polygonal), and hematoxylin vascular staining.[19,20]

When immunohistochemical stains are needed for SCLC diagnosis, the panel should include a pancytokeratin antibody such as AE1/AE3, CD56, chromogranin and synaptophysin, TTF-1, and Ki-67 (see **Fig. 2**B, C). In some cases, particularly those that are negative for TTF-1 and NE markers, p40 may be needed to exclude basaloid squamous carcinoma. In the keratin-negative setting, other tumors that need to be excluded include lymphoma (CD45 and CD20), primitive

Table 1
History of subclassification of small cell carcinoma

Kreyberg,[14] 1962	WHO,[43] 1967	1973 WP-L WHO,[15] 1981	IASLC,[16] 1998	WHO/IASLC,[18] 1999	WHO,[2] 2004
Oat cell Polygonal	Lymphocyte-like Polygonal Fusiform	Oat cell Intermediate	Pure SCLC	SCLC	SCLC
			Mixed (with large cells)		
	Other (containing squamous and glandular foci)	Combined	Combined	Combined SCLC (containing any other NSCLC component)	Combined SCLC (containing any other NSCLC component)

Abbreviations: IASLC, International Association for the Study of Lung Cancer; NSCLC, non–small cell lung carcinoma; SCLC, small cell lung carcinoma; WHO, World Health Organization; WP-L, Working Party for Therapy of Lung Cancer.
Data from Refs.[2,14–16,18,43]

Table 2
Light microscopic criteria for distinguishing small cell carcinoma and large cell carcinoma or large cell neuroendocrine carcinoma

Histologic Feature	Small Cell Carcinoma	Large Cell Carcinoma or LCNEC
Cell size	Smaller (less than diameter of 3 lymphocytes)	Larger
Nuclear/cytoplasmic ratio	Higher	Lower
Nuclear chromatin	Finely granular, uniform	Coarsely granular or vesicular Less uniform
Nucleoli	Absent or faint	Often (not always) present May be prominent or faint
Nuclear molding	Characteristic	Uncharacteristic
Fusiform shape	Common	Uncommon
Polygonal shape with ample pink cytoplasm	Uncharacteristic	Characteristic
Nuclear smear	Frequent	Uncommon
Basophilic staining of vessels and stroma	Occasional	Rare

Abbreviation: LCNEC, large cell neuroendocrine carcinoma.
  Data from Vollmer RT. The effect of cell size on the pathologic diagnosis of small and large cell carcinomas of the lung. Cancer 1982;50:1381.

neuroectodermal tumors (PNET, CD99), and melanoma (S100). TTF-1 is positive in 70% to 80% of SCLC.[21–23] Ki-67 is very helpful in distinguishing SCLC from carcinoids, because the proliferation is very high (80%–100%).[24,25]

SCLC frequently shows crush artifact in small biopsy specimens. This same artifact can occur in other tumors such as NSCLC, LCNEC, lymphoma, carcinoid tumors, and chronic inflammation. Immunohistochemistry can be very helpful in this setting. Despite the crush artifact, these tumors can readily be diagnosed with appropriate positive staining for markers such as keratin, TTF-1, chromogranin, CD56, and synaptophysin, in addition to a high proliferation rate by Ki-67.[19,24]

The tumor cells of SCLC appear larger in resected specimens than in small biopsies, owing to better fixation.[20] Thus the size of the biopsy specimen can influence the size of the tumor cell.[13,20] The larger cell size in large specimens needs to be kept in mind when reviewing this tumor in well-fixed open biopsies. Because SCLC is diagnosed by small biopsy in more than 90% of cases, most pathologists only see this tumor in small biopsies rather than in resected specimens (see **Fig. 2**D).

The distinction of SCLC from NSCLC can be difficult in approximately 5% of cases, where even expert lung cancer pathologists may disagree.[26,27] The best approach in such cases is to attempt to reach a consensus with local pathology colleagues. If a consensus cannot be reached, the case may benefit from extramural consultation with an outside expert.

SCLC very rarely occurs in a never-smoker. In this clinical setting, a thorough immunohistochemical workup should be made to exclude lymphoma, melanoma, carcinoid, and primitive neuroectodermal tumor. If the diagnosis of SCLC is confirmed, one should consider whether the tumor could be a combined SCLC with an adenocarcinoma component. *EGFR* mutations have been identified in this setting, mostly as a resistance mechanism in patients following treatment with a tyrosine kinase inhibitor.[28]

Large Cell Neuroendocrine Carcinoma

LCNEC is a high-grade non–small cell NE carcinoma classified as a variant of large cell carcinoma in the 1999 and 2004 WHO classifications.[2,18] There are 4 major categories of NE phenotypes in large cell carcinomas: (1) LCNEC with NE features by light microscopy in addition to immunohistochemistry and/or electron microscopy; (2) large cell carcinoma with NE morphology (LCNEM) but no NE differentiation by electron microscopy or immunohistochemistry; (3) large cell carcinomas with NE differentiation (LCC-NED) with no NE morphology but NE differentiation by immunohistochemistry or electron microscopy; and (4) classic large cell carcinoma that lacks both NE morphology and NE differentiation by special studies.[18,29] In surgical-resection series, LCNEC accounts for approximately 3% of cases.[30,31]

Pathology

Most LCNEC present in the peripheral lung with a mean size of 3 to 4.0 cm (range 0.9–12 cm).[32,33] The cut surface appears circumscribed with a necrotic, tan-red, cut surface.[34]

Diagnostic criteria consist of: (1) NE morphology with organoid nesting, palisading, or rosette-like structures (**Fig. 3**A); (2) high mitotic rate greater than 10 mitoses per 2 mm^2 (average 60–80 mitoses per 2 mm^2); (3) non–small cell cytologic features including large cell size, low nuclear/cytoplasmic ratio, nucleoli, or vesicular chromatin; and (4) positive immunohistochemistry for at least one NE marker such as chromogranin, CD56 or synaptophysin (see **Fig. 3**B), or electron microscopy.[2,32]

It is difficult to diagnose LCNEC in small biopsies or cytology.[30,35] Small samples are problematic because it is challenging to see the NE pattern in small tissue samples or cytology, and it can be difficult to demonstrate NE differentiation by immunohistochemistry. The recent trend of obtaining core biopsies to have sufficient tissue for molecular testing may result in more diagnoses of LCNEC in small biopsies, because the diagnostic criteria are better recognized in these specimens. However, in most cases the diagnosis of LCNEC requires a surgical lung biopsy.

The diagnosis of combined LCNEC is made when an LCNEC has components of adenocarcinoma, squamous cell carcinoma, giant cell carcinoma, and/or spindle cell carcinoma.[2,32] Adenocarcinoma is the most common additional component, but squamous cell, giant cell, or spindle cell carcinoma can also occur. When the second component is SCLC the tumor becomes a combined SCLC and LCNEC.

Immunohistochemistry and electron microscopy

The diagnosis of LCNEC requires NE differentiation to be present by immunohistochemistry or electron microscopy.[2,32] A panel of NE immunohistochemical markers should be performed including chromogranin (see **Fig. 3**B), CD56/NCAM, and synaptophysin.[29] TTF-1 will be positive in 41% to 75% of cases (see **Fig. 3**C).[21,23] With Ki-67 there is usually a high proliferation index with staining of 50% to 100% of tumor cells (see **Fig. 3**D).

Large cell carcinoma with neuroendocrine morphology The term LCNEM is used for the few large cell carcinomas that have NE morphology but no NE differentiation by immunohistochemistry or electron microscopy.[18] The few

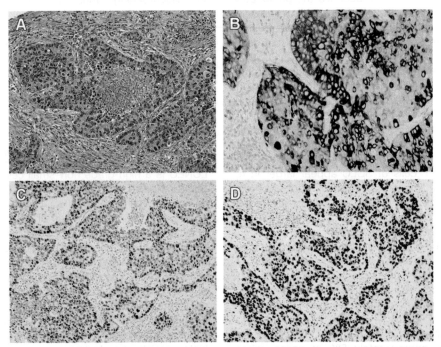

Fig. 3. LCNEC. (*A*) The tumor grows in sheets with prominent peripheral palisading and vague rosette-like structures. Several mitoses are seen. The tumor cells have abundant cytoplasm, prominent nucleoli, and an atypical mitosis (Hematoxylin and eosin ×40). (*B*) Synaptophysin strongly stains the tumor cells (Synaptophysin immunohistochemistry ×20). (*C*) TTF-1 stains many of the tumor cells (TTF-1 immunohistochemistry ×20). (*D*) Ki-67 shows a high proliferation rate, with approximately 70% staining of tumor cells (Ki-67 immunohistochemistry ×20).

published clinical data on these patients are generally similar to those for LCNEC.[33,36]

Non–small cell carcinomas with neuroendocrine differentiation Up to 10% to 20% adenocarcinomas or squamous cell carcinomas that have no NE morphology will express NE markers by immunohistochemistry, and these are called NSCLC with NE differentiation (NSCLC-NED) (see **Box 1**).[37] This expression is seen mostly in adenocarcinomas. However, this there is no proven clinical implication to this finding, either for prognosis or responsiveness to chemotherapy.[37]

Carcinoid Tumors

Pathologic features

Carcinoid tumors can present in the central or peripheral lung, with up to 40% presenting as peripheral tumors. Central carcinoids may present with an endobronchial component. Carcinoids are usually rounded tumors with a tan-yellow cut surface and an average size of 2 to 3 cm.

The histologic features of both TC and AC consist of an organoid growth pattern with uniform cytologic features consisting of a moderate amount of eosinophilic cytoplasm with an eosinophilic hue (**Fig. 4**A). Nuclei have finely granular chromatin, although in some AC it may be coarse. Nucleoli are inconspicuous in most TC, but in AC they may be more prominent.

A variety of histologic patterns may occur in both AC and TC, including spindle cell, trabecular, palisading, glandular, follicular, rosette-like, sclerosing, clear cell, and papillary patterns.[29] Tumor cells can also have unusual cytology such as oncocytic or melanocytic features. Stromal ossification or calcification can occur.

AC are defined as a carcinoid tumor with mitoses between 2 and 10 per 2-mm^2 area of viable tumor or the presence of necrosis (**Fig. 5**A).[2,29,32]

The presence of features such as pleomorphism, vascular invasion, and increased cellularity are not as helpful in separating TC from AC.[32] The necrosis in AC usually consists of small punctate foci.

A recent study of frozen sections in pulmonary carcinoid tumors showed that the most common misclassification was squamous cell carcinoma (7 of 66 cases, 11%) while lymphoma (12 of 40, 30%) and metastatic breast cancer (4 of 38, 13%) were frequently mistaken for carcinoid tumors.[38] According to a statistical analysis, the most helpful pathologic features in recognition of carcinoid versus lymphoma, squamous cell carcinoma, or metastatic breast carcinoma were central location (favoring carcinoid or squamous cell carcinoma), stromal hyalinization (favoring carcinoid), salt-and-pepper chromatin (favoring carcinoid), nuclear pleomorphism (favoring breast cancer and squamous cell carcinoma), irregular nuclear membrane (favoring breast cancer, squamous cell carcinoma, or lymphoma), and greater than 5 mitoses per 10 high-power fields (favoring squamous cell carcinoma or breast cancer).[38]

Immunohistochemistry and electron microscopy

The most useful neuroendocrine markers include chromogranin, CD56, and synaptophysin. Reports on TTF-1 expression in TC and AC are varied, with some claiming all negative[23] and others positive expression.[39] A recent report claimed that TTF-1 was expressed predominantly in peripheral rather than central carcinoids.[39] Most carcinoids stain for cytokeratins, but up to 20% to 25% may be keratin negative. Ki-67 staining shows a low proliferation rate in TC, usually less than 5% (see **Fig. 4**B) while in AC it is higher, usually between 5% and 20% (see **Fig. 5**C). The proliferation rate

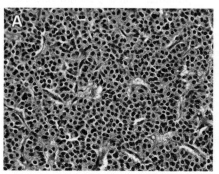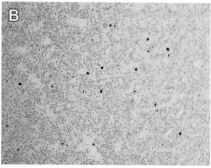

Fig. 4. Typical carcinoid. (*A*) This tumor shows an organoid nesting pattern with tumor cells that are uniform, with a moderate amount of eosinophilic cytoplasm and finely granular nuclear chromatin. No necrosis or mitoses are seen (Hematoxylin and eosin ×20). (*B*) Ki-67 shows a very low proliferation rate, with less than 5% staining of tumor cells (Ki-67 immunohistochemistry ×20).

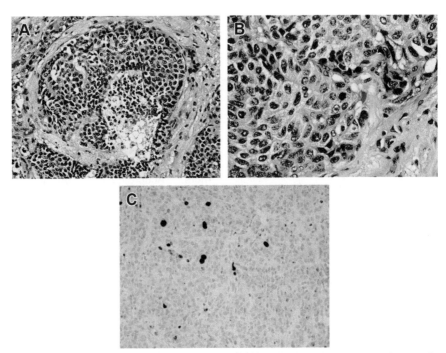

Fig. 5. Atypical carcinoid. (*A*) This tumor shows a punctate focus necrosis within sheets and nests of carcinoid tumor cells (Hematoxylin and eosin ×20). (*B*) There is a single mitosis (center) in one tumor cell. The cells have finely granular nuclear chromatin (Hematoxylin and eosin ×20). (*C*) Ki-67 shows an intermediate proliferation rate with approximately 10% staining of tumor cells (Ki-67 immunohistochemistry ×20).

can be most helpful in small crushed biopsies to separate TC or AC from LCNEC or SCLC.[24,25,40]

Dense core granules by electron microscopy are characteristic of pulmonary carcinoids, and tend to be fewer in AC than in TC.

Tumorlets and Diffuse Idiopathic Pulmonary NE Cell Hyperplasia

Tumorlets consist of nodular proliferations of NE cells that measure less than 0.5 cm in greatest diameter. Tumorlets are typically found as incidental histologic findings in lung specimens showing various inflammatory and/or fibrotic conditions such as bronchiectasis, interstitial fibrosis, chronic abscesses, or tuberculosis.

The rare condition known as DIPNECH is diagnosed when patients are found to have widespread peripheral airway NE cell hyperplasia and/or multiple tumorlets. DIPNECH is thought to represent a preinvasive lesion for carcinoid tumors, because a subset of these patients has 1 or more carcinoid tumors.[2,41,42] This lesion must be distinguished from NE cell hyperplasia and tumorlets associated with inflammation/fibrosis and local proliferations found in lung surrounding up to 75% of carcinoid tumors.

DIPNECH has 2 major presentations: (1) as a form of interstitial lung disease with airway obstruction owing to the frequent association with bronchiolar fibrosis; and (2) as multiple pulmonary nodules often mistaken for metastatic cancer. Davies and colleagues[42] reported 19 cases including 15 females and 16 nonsmokers. In this series there were 9 patients with mild interstitial lung disease such as symptomatic cough and/or dyspnea averaging 8.6 years before diagnosis, and 10 patients found incidentally to have pulmonary nodules on routine radiologic evaluation for another disorder, mostly cancer. Tumorlets and TC were found in 9 patients. Three patients had AC and 1 had multiple endocrine neoplasia type 1. Most DIPNECH patients followed an indolent clinical course, but a few progressed to severe airflow obstruction.[42]

SUMMARY

There are 4 major NE lung tumors, but the TC and AC tumors belong to a different family from the high-grade SCLC and LCNEC according to histologic, clinical, epidemiologic, and genetic features. Pathologically these tumors are primarily distinguished based on the mitotic counts, presence or absence of necrosis, and cytologic features (**Fig. 6**).

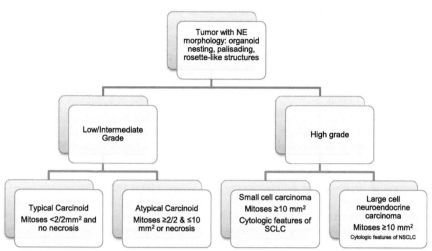

Fig. 6. Algorithm: morphologic criteria for distinguishing pulmonary neuroendocrine (NE) tumors. Tumors with NE morphology are divided into typical carcinoid, atypical carcinoid, SCLC, and LCNEC, primarily according to the presence of mitoses and necrosis. SCLC and LCNEC are separated by the cytologic features summarized in **Table 2**. NSCLC, non–small cell lung cancer.

REFERENCES

1. Travis WD. Advances in neuroendocrine lung tumors. Ann Oncol 2010;21(Suppl 7):vii65–71.
2. Travis WD, Brambilla E, Miller-Hermelink HK, et al. Pathology and genetics: tumours of the lung, pleura, thymus and heart. Lyon (France): IARC; 2004.
3. Surveillance Epidemiology, and End Results (SEER) Program. Lung cancer histologically confirmed SEER 18 registries research data plus Hurricane Katrina impacted Louisiana cases 1973–2010, November 2012; Total US County Attributes. April 2013 edition. 2013. Available at: www.seer.cancer.gov. National Cancer Institute, DCCPS, Surveillance Research Program, Surveillance Systems Branch.
4. Chen LC, Travis WD, Krug LM. Pulmonary neuroendocrine tumors: what (little) do we know? J Natl Compr Canc Netw 2006;4:623–30.
5. Clinical Lung Cancer Genome Project (CLCGP), Network Genomic Medicine (NGM). A genomics-based classification of human lung tumors. Sci Transl Med 2013;5:209ra153.
6. Fernandez-Cuesta L, Peifer M, Lu X, et al. Frequent mutations in chromatin-remodelling genes in pulmonary carcinoids. Nature communications 2014;5:3518.
7. Onuki N, Wistuba II, Travis WD, et al. Genetic changes in the spectrum of neuroendocrine lung tumors. Cancer 1999;85:600–7.
8. Hiroshima K, Iyoda A, Shibuya K, et al. Genetic alterations in early-stage pulmonary large cell neuroendocrine carcinoma. Cancer 2004;100:1190–8.
9. Iyoda A, Hiroshima K, Moriya Y, et al. Pulmonary large cell neuroendocrine carcinoma demonstrates high proliferative activity. Ann Thorac Surg 2004;77:1891–5.
10. Przygodzki RM, Finkelstein SD, Langer JC, et al. Analysis of p53, K-ras-2, and C-raf-1 in pulmonary neuroendocrine tumors. Correlation with histological subtype and clinical outcome. Am J Pathol 1996;148:1531–41.
11. Siegel R, Ma J, Zou Z, et al. Cancer statistics, 2014. CA Cancer J Clin 2014;64:9–29.
12. Govindan R, Page N, Morgensztern D, et al. Changing epidemiology of small-cell lung cancer in the United States over the last 30 years: analysis of the surveillance, epidemiologic, and end results database. J Clin Oncol 2006;24:4539–44.
13. Nicholson SA, Beasley MB, Brambilla E, et al. Small cell lung carcinoma (SCLC): a clinicopathologic study of 100 cases with surgical specimens. Am J Surg Pathol 2002;26:1184–97.
14. Kreyberg L. Histological lung cancer types. Acta Pathol Microbiol Scand Suppl 1962;157(Suppl):1–92.
15. World Health Organization, Histologic typing of lung tumours. 2nd edition. Geneva (Switzerland): World Health Organization; 1981.
16. Hirsch FR, Matthews MJ, Aisner S, et al. Histopathologic classification of small cell lung cancer. Changing concepts and terminology. Cancer 1988;62:973–7.
17. Fraire AE, Johnson EH, Yesner R, et al. Prognostic significance of histopathologic subtype and stage in small cell lung cancer. Hum Pathol 1992;23:520–8.
18. Travis WD, Colby TV, Corrin B, et al, In collaboration with Sobin LH and pathologists from 14 countries. Histological typing of lung and pleural tumors. Berlin: Springer; 1999.

19. Travis WD. Update on small cell carcinoma and its differentiation from squamous cell carcinoma and other non-small cell carcinomas. Mod Pathol 2012; 25(Suppl 1):S18–30.

20. Vollmer RT. The effect of cell size on the pathologic diagnosis of small and large cell carcinomas of the lung. Cancer 1982;50:1380–3.

21. Folpe AL, Gown AM, Lamps LW, et al. Thyroid transcription factor-1: immunohistochemical evaluation in pulmonary neuroendocrine tumors. Mod Pathol 1999;12:5–8.

22. Agoff SN, Lamps LW, Philip AT, et al. Thyroid transcription factor-1 is expressed in extrapulmonary small cell carcinomas but not in other extrapulmonary neuroendocrine tumors. Mod Pathol 2000;13:238–42.

23. Sturm N, Lantuejoul S, Laverriere MH, et al. Thyroid transcription factor 1 and cytokeratins 1, 5, 10, 14 (34betaE12) expression in basaloid and large-cell neuroendocrine carcinomas of the lung. Hum Pathol 2001;32:918–25.

24. Pelosi G, Rindi G, Travis WD, et al. Ki-67 antigen in lung neuroendocrine tumors: unraveling a role in clinical practice. J Thorac Oncol 2014;9:273–84.

25. Pelosi G, Rodriguez J, Viale G, et al. Typical and atypical pulmonary carcinoid tumor overdiagnosed as small-cell carcinoma on biopsy specimens: a major pitfall in the management of lung cancer patients. Am J Surg Pathol 2005;29:179–87.

26. Travis WD, Gal AA, Colby TV, et al. Reproducibility of neuroendocrine lung tumor classification. Hum Pathol 1998;29:272–9.

27. Roggli VL, Vollmer RT, Greenberg SD, et al. Lung cancer heterogeneity: a blinded and randomized study of 100 consecutive cases. Hum Pathol 1985; 16:569–79.

28. Shiao TH, Chang YL, Yu CJ, et al. Epidermal growth factor receptor mutations in small cell lung cancer: a brief report. J Thorac Oncol 2011;6:195–8.

29. Travis WD, Linnoila RI, Tsokos MG, et al. Neuroendocrine tumors of the lung with proposed criteria for large-cell neuroendocrine carcinoma. An ultrastructural, immunohistochemical, and flow cytometric study of 35 cases. Am J Surg Pathol 1991;15:529–53.

30. Travis WD. Neuroendocrine lung tumors. Path Case Reviews 2006;11:235–42.

31. Iyoda A, Hiroshima K, Baba M, et al. Pulmonary large cell carcinomas with neuroendocrine features are high-grade neuroendocrine tumors. Ann Thorac Surg 2002;73:1049–54.

32. Travis WD, Rush W, Flieder DB, et al. Survival analysis of 200 pulmonary neuroendocrine tumors with clarification of criteria for atypical carcinoid and its separation from typical carcinoid. Am J Surg Pathol 1998;22:934–44.

33. Iyoda A, Hiroshima K, Toyozaki T, et al. Clinical characterization of pulmonary large cell neuroendocrine carcinoma and large cell carcinoma with neuroendocrine morphology. Cancer 2001;91:1992–2000.

34. Oshiro Y, Kusumoto M, Matsuno Y, et al. CT findings of surgically resected large cell neuroendocrine carcinoma of the lung in 38 patients. AJR Am J Roentgenol 2004;182:87–91.

35. Hiroshima K, Abe S, Ebihara Y, et al. Cytological characteristics of pulmonary large cell neuroendocrine carcinoma. Lung Cancer 2005;48:331–7.

36. Zacharias J, Nicholson AG, Ladas GP, et al. Large cell neuroendocrine carcinoma and large cell carcinomas with neuroendocrine morphology of the lung: prognosis after complete resection and systematic nodal dissection. Ann Thorac Surg 2003;75:348–52.

37. Ionescu DN, Treaba D, Gilks CB, et al. Nonsmall cell lung carcinoma with neuroendocrine differentiation - an entity of no clinical or prognostic significance. Am J Surg Pathol 2007;31:26–32.

38. Gupta R, Dastane A, McKenna RJ Jr, et al. What can we learn from the errors in the frozen section diagnosis of pulmonary carcinoid tumors? An evidence-based approach. Hum Pathol 2009;40: 1–9.

39. Du EZ, Goldstraw P, Zacharias J, et al. TTF-1 expression is specific for lung primary in typical and atypical carcinoids: TTF-1-positive carcinoids are predominantly in peripheral location. Hum Pathol 2004;35:825–31.

40. Rindi G, Klersy C, Inzani F, et al. Grading the neuroendocrine tumors of the lung: an evidence-based proposal. Endocr Relat Cancer 2014;21:1–16.

41. Nassar AA, Jaroszewski DE, Helmers RA, et al. Diffuse idiopathic pulmonary neuroendocrine cell hyperplasia: a systematic overview. Am J Respir Crit Care Med 2011;184:8–16.

42. Davies SJ, Gosney JR, Hansell DM, et al. Diffuse idiopathic pulmonary neuroendocrine cell hyperplasia: an under-recognised spectrum of disease. Thorax 2007;62:248–52.

43. World Health Organization. Histological typing of lung tumours. Geneva (Switzerland): World Health Organization; 1967.

Clinical Presentation and Evaluation of Neuroendocrine Tumors of the Lung

Frank C. Detterbeck, MD

KEYWORDS

- Carcinoid tumors • Bronchopulmonary carcinoid tumors • Neuroendocrine tumors of the lung
- Clinical presentation

KEY POINTS

- Carcinoid tumors can usually be reliably clinically diagnosed (ie, either a smooth endobronchial lesion or an asymptomatic round parenchymal nodule).
- Biopsy confirmation of a carcinoid tumor is usually unnecessary and distinction of typical versus atypical carcinoid tumor by biopsy is usually unreliable.
- Clinical distinction of typical versus atypical carcinoid tumors can be predicted based on age, tumor location, and nodal size, which guide further staging tests.
- Large cell neuroendocrine lung cancer presents similarly to non-small cell lung cancer and the clinical evaluation is the same.
- Small cell lung cancer is strongly predicted by rapid progression of symptoms and a bulky central mediastinal tumor.

INTRODUCTION

Neuroendocrine tumors (NETs) of the lung all display neuroendocrine granules on microscopic examination; however, these tumors cover a wide spectrum. This includes demographic features, epidemiologic aspects, the clinical and radiographic presentations, as well as the prognosis and treatment. In keeping with this, the approach to these cases is varied. This article focuses on the clinical and radiographic presentation and uses these to build a clinical approach to the evaluation of patients.

CLINICAL PRESENTATION
Epidemiology

Patients with bronchopulmonary carcinoid tumors are younger than patients with non-small cell lung cancer (NSCLC), with median ages of 48 and 70, respectively.[1–3] There is a broad age distribution and a relatively equal gender distribution.[3] Patients with an atypical carcinoid (AC) tumor are older than those with a typical carcinoid (TC) tumor (<10% of carcinoid tumors are AC in patients <30 years old, gradually increasing to ~25% in those older than age 60).[3–6] These tumors seem to not be related to smoking.[3,7]

In general, patients with small cell lung cancer (SCLC) and large cell neuroendocrine lung cancer (LCNEC) have the demographic distribution of SCLC and NSCLC patients. The median age is around 70 and the gender distribution is relatively equal in North America.[8,9] LCNEC is rare, accounting for less than 1% of pulmonary NETs.[9] Smoking is so strongly associated with SCLC that the diagnosis must be questioned in a nonsmoker.[10–12]

The author has nothing to disclose.
Yale Thoracic Surgery, Yale University, PO Box 208062, New Haven, CT 06520-8062, USA
E-mail address: frank.detterbeck@yale.edu

Thorac Surg Clin 24 (2014) 267–276
http://dx.doi.org/10.1016/j.thorsurg.2014.04.002

Abbreviations	
AC	Atypical carcinoid
CT	Computed tomography imaging
LCNEC	Large cell neuroendocrine lung cancer
MET	Mucoepidermoid tumor
MRI	Magnetic resonance imaging
NET	Neuroendocrine tumor
NSCLC	Non-small cell lung cancer
PET	Positron emission tomography
SCLC	Small cell lung cancer
TC	Typical carcinoid
TTNA	Transthoracic-needle aspiration
5-HIAA	5-hydroxyindoleacetic acid

LCNEC also seems to be strongly correlated with smoking, although not as exclusively as SCLC.[13–15]

Symptoms

Central carcinoid tumors often present with symptoms related to airway obstruction (cough, recurrent pneumonia, wheezing, and hemoptysis) and many patients are treated for prolonged periods for asthma or infection.[1,3,16,17] On the other hand, peripheral carcinoid tumors are usually discovered incidentally in patients without symptoms.

Patients with SCLC are almost always symptomatic, typically with rapid progression of symptoms consistent with the rapid growth of these tumors. Common symptoms include systemic complaints (weight loss and fatigue) as well as those due to bulky central disease (cough dyspnea, chest pain, hemoptysis, and hoarseness).[18] The clinical presentation of LCNEC is less well defined but, in general, parallels that of NSCLC. Although patients with NSCLC may be asymptomatic, cough, hemoptysis, dyspnea, persistent pneumonia, chest pain, weight loss, and fatigue are common.[19] The progression of symptoms with LCNEC generally lasts months, instead of weeks as in SCLC.

Endocrine Syndromes

Carcinoid tumors

Carcinoid syndrome (episodic flushing and diarrhea) is distinctly rare in patients with bronchopulmonary carcinoid tumors, occurring in less than 1% of patients at presentation and in less than 5% during the subsequent course.[2–4,9,20–28] However, studies suggest that mild complaints of diarrhea or flushing may be elicited in approximately 10% of patients.[16,29] True carcinoid syndrome is almost exclusively seen in patients with liver metastases.[24,30] These data clearly refute the frequently cited speculation that carcinoid syndrome is seen when carcinoid tumors drain into the systemic, as opposed to the portal, circulation. Instead, development of carcinoid syndrome may be related to tumor burden.

Although mild elevation of serotonin or its urinary metabolite, 5-hydroxyindoleacetic acid (5-HIAA), have been reported by some investigators,[16] others have found these only rarely abnormal.[7,29] Routine assessment of these laboratory tests does not seem to be useful and is not recommended.[3,7]

Nevertheless, rare cases of therapeutic interventions have been reported, including initiation of chemotherapy precipitating carcinoid crisis (a life-threatening condition involving flushing, confusion, coma, and either hypotension or hypertension).[31] This is treated by administration of somatostatin.[31–34]

A more frequent endocrine syndrome seen in patients with bronchopulmonary carcinoid tumors is Cushing syndrome, occurring in approximately 4% of patients.[2,16,31,35–38] Bronchial carcinoids account for the most common source of ectopic Cushing syndrome and a search for such a tumor is warranted.[31] Most of these patients have small localized tumors, often only visible on CT.[38] These are usually peripheral tumors. About 80% are TC tumors.[2,39,40] In most patients the syndrome resolves after resection.[36,38,41]

Other endocrine syndromes are rarely reported.[31] These include several cases of acromegaly, which resolved after resection.[2,31,42–44] A case of a patient with elevated parathyroid hormone resulting from a metastatic pulmonary carcinoid tumor was reported.[45] Cardiac valvular disease attributed to a carcinoid tumor has been extremely rarely reported and these involved the right (not left) heart valves.[30]

SCLC or LCNEC

There is a well-known association of SCLC with various paraneoplastic syndromes, which are described in more detail by Ferone.[46] These include the syndrome of inappropriate antidiuretic hormone, hyponatremia, ectopic corticotropin production, and Eaton-Lambert syndrome. LCNECs are not generally associated with paraneoplastic syndromes, although owing to the rarity of these tumors this is less well defined.

RADIOGRAPHIC PRESENTATION
Central Carcinoid Tumors

Approximately 70% of carcinoid tumors present as central tumors.[2–5,16,25,27,28,35,37,41,47,48] Central is not precisely defined but usually means that it is visible by bronchoscopy. Most are located in segmental bronchi (**Fig. 1**), with a predilection for the right middle lobe and the lingula.[3] Carcinoid tumors occurring in more central airways are relatively uncommon.

The radiographic appearance of central carcinoid tumors is not distinctive. There is often atelectasis of a portion of the lung.[1] Central carcinoid tumors are predominantly TC.[3] Node enlargement is less common; however, it may be difficult to distinguish an adjacent node from a central mass and obstructive pneumonia may cause reactive node enlargement. It is important to perform a CT scan with contrast to better define the anatomy.[3]

Peripheral Carcinoid Tumors

The radiographic features of a central or peripheral carcinoid tumor on a chest CT scan are usually characteristic. A peripheral carcinoid tumor generally appears as a sharply demarcated, round, homogeneous mass, situated somewhat deeply in the lung. A CT scan with vascular contrast is helpful to identify hilar node enlargement. This is important because approximately one-third of peripheral carcinoid tumors are AC, which are more likely to show node involvement.[3]

Metabolic Imaging for Carcinoid Tumors

The role of positron emission tomography (PET) imaging for carcinoid tumors is not well-defined. In general, the degree of PET uptake is low but there are conflicting data on the detection of pulmonary carcinoids by PET. The reported sensitivity of PET ranges from 14% to 100% for diagnosis of the primary tumor as malignant in several small studies (7, 13, and 16 subjects).[49–51] The sensitivity may be higher with AC compared with TC (80% vs 73%).[51] The reported data do not permit calculation of specificity, false-negative or false-positive rates, for diagnosis of the primary tumor. These studies have involved a high proportion of peripherally located carcinoids (57%–81%), which have a slightly higher proportion of AC.[49–51]

Although ^{111}In-labeled octreotide imaging is commonly used with abdominal carcinoids, the impact in bronchopulmonary carcinoid tumors is limited. About 35% of bronchial carcinoids are somatostatin receptor negative[52] and the intensity is usually weak and similar to what is seen in areas of inflammation (octreotide binds to white blood cell receptors). Furthermore, octreotide scans are positive in most subjects with NSCLC and SCLC, and in subjects with lymphoma, sarcoidosis, granuloma, and pneumonia.[52,53] Nevertheless, small studies (8–28 subjects) have reported 81% to 100% sensitivity for detecting a bronchopulmonary carcinoid tumor,[52,54,55] with a 19% false-negative rate.[52] Specificity and false-positive rates are not available from the reported data.

SCLC

Most patients with SCLC present with bulky hilar and mediastinal lymphadenopathy. The primary tumor is usually central, often overshadowed by the mediastinal involvement. A peripheral primary tumor is distinctly rare. Most patients with SCLC have distant metastases at the time of presentation.[8] Consistent with the high degree of metabolic activity, SCLC are highly PET avid, and PET is indicated for staging (unless distant metastases are already obvious).[56]

LCNEC

LCNEC typically are observed to be radiographically similar to NSCLC. There is usually a peripheral parenchymal mass, without or with (less common) nodal enlargement.[13–15] However, most reports of LCNEC involve resected tumors, likely reflecting that it is often difficult to identify

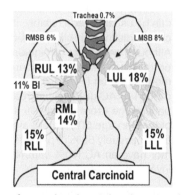

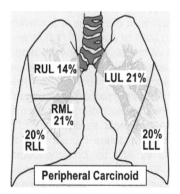

Fig. 1. Distribution of central and peripheral carcinoids (TC and AC). Values represent an average taken from studies of more than 50 subjects from 1975 to 2007.[4,7,22,24,47,61–63,66] BI, bronchus intermedius; LLL, left lower lobe; LMSB, left main stem bronchus; LUL, left upper lobe; RLL, right lower lobe; RML, right middle lobe; RMSB, right main stem bronchus; RLL, right lower lobe. (*From* Detterbeck FC. Management of carcinoid tumors. Ann Thorac Surg 2010;89(3):999; with permission.)

an LCNEC from a small biopsy. Thus the reported radiographic presentation may be skewed toward less advanced tumors.

CLINICAL APPROACH TO PATIENTS
Central Carcinoid Tumors

Clinical diagnosis
Most patients with a central carcinoid tumor present in a way that allows a clinical diagnosis to be reliably made without a tissue biopsy. Symptoms of segmental or lobar airway obstruction, usually ongoing for a long time in a young patient (younger than age 40) is suggestive of a carcinoid tumor. When the CT scan or bronchoscopy demonstrates a focal, smooth endobronchial tumor in a lobar or segmental bronchus (with or without an extrabronchial component) there is little doubt. Squamous cell carcinoma is uncommon in younger patients and appears friable on bronchoscopy and less clearly demarcated on CT scan. Adenoid cystic carcinoma usually occurs in the trachea (~90%) and is also less focal.[57] The presentation of a mucoepidermoid tumors (METs) is very similar (demographics, symptoms, and location) but these are 10 to 20 times less common and are managed in essentially the same manner.[1]

Diagnostic interventions
In patients suspected of having a central tumor, a CT scan should be done with intravenous contrast to assess the extent of the tumor and the relationship to surrounding vessels. The vast majority of central carcinoid tumors are visible with bronchoscopy and have a characteristic appearance: smooth and rounded, red or reddish-brown, and are often covered by bronchial mucosa. This essentially rules out other airway tumors (except METs) and is helpful to further confirm the clinical diagnosis. Biopsy is well-documented as safe (self-limited bleeding in 1.4% and major bleeding in 0.3%, all from one older study).[1,58] However, a diagnosis is achieved in only about 70% to 80% of cases.[7,58,59] Furthermore, in about 10% of cases, an erroneous diagnosis is made (usually SCLC or squamous carcinoma),[1] underscoring the importance of the clinical diagnosis in evaluating pathologic findings. Establishing a diagnosis of carcinoid tumor seems more difficult with AC in most studies.[37,41,60–62] Furthermore, the ability to define the subtype of carcinoid tumor (TC vs AC) by bronchoscopic biopsy is only about 40%.[37,41,60,62] This is not surprising because about 2 mm^2 of well-preserved tumor is needed for adequate assessment.

Staging considerations
In most patients with a central carcinoid tumor and a typical presentation, a clinical diagnosis of carcinoid tumor can be reliably made, sometimes confirmed by biopsy. However, in most cases, the ability to distinguish TC from AC remains in question. This is important because it influences further staging considerations and treatment strategy. If there is no node enlargement (N1 or N2), most patients have a TC (**Fig. 2**). This is even more true if they are young. In such cases there is little role for invasive mediastinal staging or for imaging investigations for distant metastases because the incidence of occult tumor spread is low and resection is indicated even in the face of mediastinal node (pN2) involvement of a TC. A PET scan is rarely useful in distinguishing the tumor from a more metabolically active tumor (NSCLC or SCLC). If there is node enlargement, invasive mediastinal staging seems to be appropriate, although the optimal treatment approach for a central N2-positive AC is unclear and may still involve primary resection.[3,58]

Peripheral Carcinoid Tumors

Clinical diagnosis
Peripheral carcinoid tumors are invariably sharply demarcated, smooth, and typically round. If previous films are available, they are found to grow slowly. They have little metabolic activity, so there is little value in a PET scan other than to rule out another disease. Unless there is an unusual history or findings on the abdominal portion of the chest CT scan, it can be reliably assumed that a peripheral carcinoid tumor is a primary pulmonary carcinoid tumor and there is no need to search for another source. Ectopic corticotropin production is rare but a virtually pathognomonic symptom that a peripheral nodule is a carcinoid tumor.[39–41] Thus most peripheral carcinoid tumors can be diagnosed as such on clinical grounds by an experienced clinician with a high degree of reliability.

Although a clinical diagnosis of carcinoid tumor can be usually made reliably, it is much more difficult to distinguish clinically between TC and AC. Although peripheral carcinoids have a higher proportion of AC than central carcinoids, a TC is still more common (~70% TC, ~30% AC). The proportion of AC gradually increases with increasing patient age (from about 5% if <age 25 to 25% if older than age 50). If there are nodal metastases, approximately 50% of patients with a carcinoid tumor have an AC (40% with N1 and 75% with N2 involvement, see **Fig. 2**).

Diagnostic interventions
A transthoracic-needle aspiration (TTNA) is the most common diagnostic intervention for a peripheral nodule. However, the ability to secure the diagnosis of a carcinoid tumor is only about

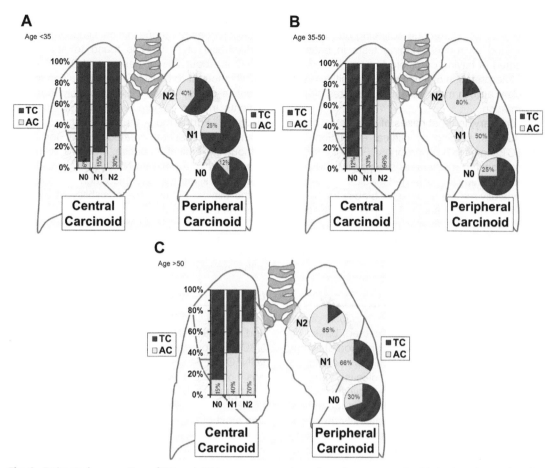

Fig. 2. Estimated proportion of TC and AC tumors among bronchopulmonary carcinoids by location and patho-logic nodal status. (*A*) Age <35. (*B*) Age 35–50. (*C*) Age >50. Results are a rough estimate based on age distribu-tion, proportion of TC versus AC tumors, and rate of node involvement.

40% (range 20%–80%).[24,26,63–65] The ability to distinguish between carcinoid tumor subtypes by TTNA is even lower.[64,65] Therefore, if the clinical presentation and appearance strongly suggest a carcinoid tumor, a TTNA may not be worthwhile and can be misleading. The clinical diagnosis is often the most reliable and important step in the process of patient evaluation.

Unfortunately, intraoperative frozen section diagnosis is also notoriously difficult. A diagnosis of carcinoid tumor is made on frozen section in only about 50%.[7,22,63,66] About half of the remainder are interpreted to be either SCLC or NSCLC, and a variety of benign conditions in the other half. Thus the clinical diagnosis established preoperatively should weigh heavily in the inter-pretation of a frozen section result and probably renders the frozen section unnecessary in many cases. These data make it highly questionable whether a frozen section can distinguish between TC and AC, although data defining this is not available.

Staging considerations

A negative clinical evaluation seems likely to be sufficiently reliable without further imaging for distant metastases,[58] although this has not been well-defined. A study of 40 central and peripheral carcinoid tumors found that nodal assessment by CT had a sensitivity of 67%, specificity of 97%, and a 6% false-negative and a 20% false-positive rate.[63] Taken together with the data for NSCLC in general, this suggests that invasive staging (mediastinoscopy) is indicated if node enlargement is seen by CT.

There are no data that define the reliability of PET for staging of carcinoid tumors, either at distant sites or in the mediastinum. However, the generally lower degree of PET activity for carcinoid tumors compared with NSCLC and that, in NSCLC, PET carries a false-positive and a false-negative rate in the mediastinum of about 15% to 20%,[67] it is likely that PET carries a high false-negative rate in carcinoid tumors. The reliability of octreotide scanning for staging has also not been defined (see previous discussion). Thus neither PET nor octreotide scanning can be recommended as routine staging tests in patients suspected of having carcinoid tumors. If they are done, interpretation of a negative or positive result is unclear and, in most instances, requires biopsy confirmation.

In summary, in most cases of suspected carcinoid tumors, staging by clinical evaluation and chest CT seems to be appropriate. Further imaging for unsuspected metastases seems unwarranted. Suspicious areas (eg, enlarged mediastinal nodes) will generally require an invasive biopsy for confirmation. In general, surgical biopsy (mediastinoscopy) is preferred over a needle technique (ie, endobronchial ultrasound) to confirm carcinoid tumor as well as to reliably differentiate between TC and AC.

SCLC

In most patients with SCLC, the diagnosis of this cell type is usually strongly suspected, based on age and risk factors, a rapid progression of symptoms, and the typical radiographic appearance of bulky central and mediastinal disease (**Fig. 3**). This is usually sufficiently reliable to initiate the process of staging and evaluation for treatment, although there are no data that quantify the accuracy of the clinical diagnosis. Furthermore, because treatment is usually nonsurgical, an invasive diagnostic procedure will be necessary.

In patients suspected to have SCLC, the diagnosis should be obtained by whatever method is judged to be easiest, including sputum cytology, thoracentesis, fine-needle aspiration, or bronchoscopy.[68] The diagnosis can generally be readily achieved but the sensitivity is higher with biopsies involving histologic specimens instead of cytology.[69] However, it is important to keep in mind the possibility of an erroneous cell type diagnosis if it does not fit the clinical situation. Overall, a diagnosis of NSCLC is found to actually be SCLC in about 2% of cases, and 9% of cases initially thought to be SCLC are NSCLC on subsequent re-biopsy (these cases probably represent patients in whom there was a suspicion of an error).[68,69] Furthermore, there are many anecdotal examples of patients treated initially for SCLC without the typical response, who are eventually found to have a different NET (ie, AC or LCNEC). Therefore, if the microscopic diagnosis does not fit the clinical picture, the possibility of an error must be considered.

Staging of SCLC is achieved by imaging studies (CT of chest or abdomen, brain MRI, and PET).[56] There is rarely a need to confirm an imaging finding with a biopsy.

LCNEC

In general, LCNEC tumors present just like NSCLC and do lend themselves to a clinical diagnosis of NSCLC. However, there is nothing specific for LCNEC that lends itself to making a clinical diagnosis of this entity.

A further problem is that it is difficult to diagnose LCNEC from only preoperative biopsy specimens and most of these tumors are identified only after resection.[70] When a preoperative diagnosis was available, the tumor was often thought to be an AC, poorly differentiated carcinoma, or SCLC with an intermediate cell type.[70,71] Complicating matters further is that there is significant interobserver variability in classifying resected tumors as either SCLC or LCNEC. In a study of 170 resected cases and nine thoracic expert pathologists, the correlation was only fair (kappa = 0.4).[72] It is unclear how much difference this makes clinically. The *American College of Chest Physicians Lung*

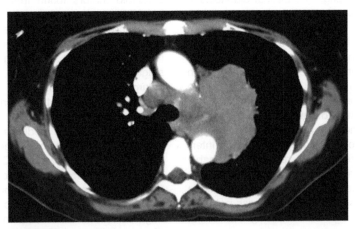

Fig. 3. CT of a patient with SCLC.

Cancer Guidelines[56] recommend resection of an SCLC tumor that appears resectable; the same recommendation can be made for LCNEC. Further details are unclear, such as whether to administer chemotherapy before or after, what type of chemotherapy, and whether the approach should be different for SCLC and NSCLC.

The staging evaluation for a patient with LCNEC should be the same as for any patient with NSCLC (or, for that matter, a patient with early stage SCLC).[56,67] Therefore, it is of little consequence that a preoperative diagnosis of LCNEC usually cannot be made (either from clinical features or biopsies). These patients should be approached as is standard for any other NSCLC patient.

SUMMARY

Although NETs can be grouped together based on neuroendocrine granules, this creates a wide spectrum of entities. To an extent, these belong in two groups: TC or AC and SCLC or LCNEC. The TC or AC tumors are less aggressive, often occur in younger patients, and seem not to be related to smoking. Both SCLC and LCNEC are aggressive and occur mainly in older patients with a history of smoking.

The clinical presentation of carcinoid tumors is characteristic, although it involves two distinct forms: a central airway tumor or a peripheral parenchymal lesion. The central carcinoid tumors cause typical airway obstructive symptoms, usually present in younger patients, and have a characteristic bronchoscopic appearance. The peripheral tumors are usually asymptomatic, occur in middle-aged individuals, and have a characteristic radiographic appearance (round and well-demarcated). SCLC also has a characteristic presentation, involving a bulky central mass and significant rapidly progressive symptoms. On the other hand, there are no features that distinguish LCNEC from other types of NSCLC.

It is important to establish a clinical diagnosis for carcinoid tumors. Although a bronchoscopic biopsy is safe and often achieves a diagnosis in central carcinoid tumors, there remains a substantial rate of misdiagnoses. Furthermore, the distinction between TC and AC is notoriously unreliable except in a resected specimen. The same is true of peripheral carcinoids and either TTNA or frozen section assessment. Therefore, the clinical diagnosis of either TC or AC must continue to be weighed heavily when biopsy results are interpreted.

An assessment of the likelihood of TC versus AC can be made from the patient's age, type of presentation, and clinical stage. If there is node enlargement, a mediastinoscopy is generally indicated to establish the stage, diagnosis of TC versus AC, and to rule out other cancers. A clinical evaluation is generally sufficient to evaluate for distant metastases. Routine imaging with PET or octreotide has a significant chance of being misleading.

The clinical diagnosis and tissue confirmation of SCLC are generally straightforward. However, if a tissue diagnosis of SCLC is made in a patient in whom the clinical presentation is atypical, the possibility of an erroneous diagnosis must be considered. LCNEC is rarely diagnosed before resection, either on a clinical or microscopic basis. However, these cases present like other NSCLC and should be approached from a staging standpoint the same way.

Knowledge of the clinical characteristics of NETs defines an approach to the evaluation of patients, which is likely to lead to an efficient work-up and avoidance of errors in diagnosis or management.

REFERENCES

1. Detterbeck FC. Management of carcinoid tumors. Ann Thorac Surg 2010;89(3):998–1005.
2. Bertelsen S, Aasted A, Lund C, et al. Bronchial carcinoid tumours: a clinicopathologic study of 82 cases. Scand J Thorac Cardiovasc Surg 1985;19:105–11.
3. Paladugu RR, Benfield JR, Pak HY, et al. Bronchopulmonary Kulchitzky cell carcinomas: a new classification scheme for typical and atypical carcinoids. Cancer 1985;55:1301–11.
4. Hurt R, Bates M. Carcinoid tumours of the bronchus: a 33 year experience. Thorax 1984;39:617–23.
5. El Jamal M, Nicholson AG, Goldstraw P. The feasibility of conservative resection for carcinoid tumours: is pneumonectomy ever necessary for uncomplicated cases? Eur J Cardiothorac Surg 2000;18(3):301–6.
6. Govindan R, Page N, Morgensztern D, et al. Changing epidemiology of small-cell lung cancer in the United States over the last 30 years: analysis of the surveillance, epidemiologic, and end results database. J Clin Oncol 2006;24(28):4539–44.
7. Gustafsson BI, Kidd M, Chan A, et al. Bronchopulmonary neuroendocrine tumors. Cancer 2008;113(1):5–21.
8. Auerbach O, Garfinkel L. The changing pattern of lung carcinoma. Cancer 1991;68:1973–7.
9. Morabia A, Wynder EL. Cigarette smoking and lung cancer cell types. Cancer 1991;68:2074–8.

10. Vincent RG, Pickren JW, Lane WW, et al. The changing histopathology of lung cancer: a review of 1682 cases. Cancer 1977;39:1647–55.

11. Veronesi G, Morandi U, Alloisio M, et al. Large cell neuroendocrine carcinoma of the lung: a retrospective analysis of 144 surgical cases. Lung Cancer 2006;53(1):111–5.

12. Asamura H, Kameya T, Matsuno Y, et al. Neuroendocrine neoplasms of the lung: a prognostic spectrum. J Clin Oncol 2006;24(1):70–6.

13. Akata S, Okada S, Maeda J, et al. Computed tomographic findings of large cell neuroendocrine carcinoma of the lung. Clin Imaging 2007;31(6):379–84.

14. Soga J, Yakuwa Y. Bronchopulmonary carcinoids: an analysis of 1875 reported cases with special reference to a comparison between typical carcinoids and atypical varieties. Ann Thorac Cardiovasc Surg 1999;5:211–9.

15. Hage R, de la Riviere AB, Seldenrijk CA, et al. Update in pulmonary carcinoid tumors: a review article. Ann Surg Oncol 2003;10(6):697–704.

16. Kiser AC, Detterbeck FC. Carcinoid and mucoepidermoid tumors. In: Detterbeck FC, Rivera MP, Socinski MA, et al, editors. Diagnosis and treatment of lung cancer: an evidence-based guide for the practicing clinician. Philadelphia: W. B. Saunders; 2001. p. 379–93.

17. Chute C, Greenberg E, Baron J, et al. Presenting conditions of 1539 population-based lung cancer patients by cell type and stage in New Hampshire and Vermont. Cancer 1985;56:2107–11.

18. Huhti E, Sutinen S, Reinilä A, et al. Lung cancer in a defined geographical area: history and histological types. Thorax 1980;35:660–7.

19. Attar S, Miller JE, Hankins J, et al. Bronchial adenoma: a review of 51 patients. Ann Thorac Surg 1985;40:126–32.

20. Rea F, Binda R, Spreafico G, et al. Bronchial carcinoids: a review of 60 patients. Ann Thorac Surg 1989;47:412–4.

21. McCaughan BC, Martini N, Bains MS. Bronchial carcinoids: review of 124 cases. J Thorac Cardiovasc Surg 1985;89(1):8–17.

22. Mårtensson H, Böttcher G, Hambraeus G, et al. Bronchial carcinoids: an analysis of 91 cases. World J Surg 1987;11:356–64.

23. Fink G, Krelbaum T, Yellin A, et al. Pulmonary carcinoid: presentation, diagnosis, and outcome in 142 cases in Israel and review of 640 cases from the literature. Chest 2001;119(6):1647–51.

24. Daddi N, Ferolla P, Urbani M, et al. Surgical treatment of neuroendocrine tumors of the lung. Eur J Cardiothorac Surg 2004;26(4):813–7.

25. Cardillo G, Sera F, Di Martino M, et al. Bronchial carcinoid tumors: nodal status and long-term survival after resection. Ann Thorac Surg 2004;77(5):1781–5.

26. Garcia-Yuste M, Matilla JM, Cueto A, et al. Typical and atypical carcinoid tumours: analysis of the experience of the Spanish Multi-centric Study of Neuroendocrine Tumours of the Lung. Eur J Cardiothorac Surg 2007;31(2):192–7.

27. Rea F, Rizzardi G, Zuin A, et al. Outcome and surgical strategy in bronchial carcinoid tumors: single institution experience with 252 patients. Eur J Cardiothorac Surg 2007;31(2):186–91.

28. Kurul IC, Topcu S, Tastepe I, et al. Surgery in bronchial carcinoids: experience with 83 patients. Eur J Cardiothorac Surg 2002;21(5):883–7.

29. Harpole DH Jr, Feldman JM, Buchanan S, et al. Bronchial carcinoid tumors: a retrospective analysis of 126 patients. Ann Thorac Surg 1992;54:50–5.

30. Ricci C, Patrassi N, Massa R, et al. Carcinoid syndrome in bronchial adenoma. Am J Surg 1973;126:671–7.

31. Davila D, Dunn W, Tazelaar H, et al. Bronchial carcinoid tumors. Mayo Clin Proc 1993;68:795–803.

32. Marsh HM, Martin JK, Kvols LK, et al. Carcinoid crisis during anesthesia: successful treatment with a somatostatin analogue. Anesthesiology 1987;66:89–91.

33. Granberg D, Eriksson B, Wilander E, et al. Experience in treatment of metastatic pulmonary carcinoid tumors. Ann Oncol 2001;12(10):1383–91.

34. Maroun J, Walter K, Kvols L, et al. Guidelines for the diagnosis and management of carcinoid tumours, part 1: the gastrointestinal tract. A statement from a Canadian National Carcinoid Expert Group. Curr Oncol 2006;13(2):67–76.

35. Ducrocq X, Thomas P, Massard G, et al. Operative risk and prognostic factors of typical bronchial carcinoid tumors. Ann Thorac Surg 1998;65:1410–4.

36. Wilkins EW Jr, Grillo HC, Moncure AC, et al. Changing times in surgical management of bronchopulmonary carcinoid tumor. Ann Thorac Surg 1984;38:339–44.

37. Warren WH, Faber LP, Gould VE. Neuroendocrine neoplasms of the lung. J Thorac Cardiovasc Surg 1989;98(3):321–32.

38. Limper AH, Carpenter PC, Scheithauer B, et al. The Cushing syndrome induced by bronchial carcinoid tumors. Ann Intern Med 1992;117:209–14.

39. Pass HI, Doppman JL, Nieman L, et al. Management of the ectopic ACTH syndrome due to thoracic carcinoids. Ann Thorac Surg 1990;50(1):52–7.

40. Shrager JB, Wright CD, Wain JC, et al. Bronchopulmonary carcinoid tumors associated with Cushing's syndrome: a more aggressive variant of typical carcinoid. J Thorac Cardiovasc Surg 1997;114(3):367–75.

41. Marty-Ané CH, Costes V, Pujol JL, et al. Carcinoid tumors of the lung: do atypical features require

aggressive management? Ann Thorac Surg 1995; 59:78–83.

42. Garcia-Luna PP, Leal-Cerro A, Montero C, et al. A rare cause of acromegaly: ectopic production of growth hormone-releasing factor by a bronchial carcinoid tumor. Surg Neurol 1987;27:563–8.

43. Carroll D, Delahunt J, Teague C, et al. Resolution of acromegaly after removal of a bronchial carcinoid shown to secrete growth hormone releasing factor. Aust NZ J Med 1987;17:63–7.

44. Sönksen PH, Ayres AB, Braimbridge M, et al. Acromegaly caused by pulmonary carcinoid tumours. Clin Endocrinol 1976;5:503–13.

45. Docherty HM, Heath DA. Multiple forms of parathyroid hormone-like proteins in a human tumour. J Mol Endocrinol 1989;2:11–20.

46. Ferone D. Neuroendocrine tumors and endocrine syndromes. Thorac Surg Clin 2014;24(3).

47. Schreurs JM, Westermann CJ, van den Bosch JM, et al. A twenty-five-year follow-up of ninety-three resected typical carcinoid tumors of the lung. J Thorac Cardiovasc Surg 1992;104(5):1470–5.

48. Schrevens L, Vansteenkiste J, Deneffe G, et al. Clinical-radiological presentation and outcome of surgically treated pulmonary carcinoid tumours: a long-term single institution experience. Lung Cancer 2004;43(1):39–45.

49. Kruger S, Buck AK, Blumstein NM, et al. Use of integrated FDG PET/CT imaging in pulmonary carcinoid tumours. J Intern Med 2006;260(6): 545–50.

50. Erasmus J, McAdams H, Patz E, et al. Evaluation of primary pulmonary carcinoid tumors using FDG PET. AJR Am J Roentgenol 1998;170(5): 1369–73.

51. Daniels CE, Lowe VJ, Aubry MC, et al. The utility of fluorodeoxyglucose positron emission tomography in the evaluation of carcinoid tumors presenting as pulmonary nodules. Chest 2007;131(1): 255–60.

52. Granberg D, Sundin A, Janson ET, et al. Octreoscan in patients with bronchial carcinoid tumours. Clin Endocrinol 2003;59(6):793–9.

53. Lau SK, Johnson DS, Coel MN. Imaging of non-small-cell lung cancer with indium-111 pentetreotide. Clin Nucl Med 2000;25(1):24–8.

54. Yellin A, Zwas S, Rozenman J, et al. Experience with somatostatin receptor scintigraphy in the management of pulmonary carcinoid tumors. Isr Med Assoc J 2005;1(11):712–6.

55. Musi M, Carbone RG, Bertocchi C, et al. Bronchial carcinoid tumours: a study on clinicopathological features and role of octreotide scintigraphy. Lung Cancer 1998;22(2):97–102.

56. Jett J, Schild S, Kesler K, et al. Treatment of small cell lung cancer: Diagnosis and management of lung cancer, 3rd ed: American College of Chest Physicians evidence-based clinical practice guidelines. Chest 2013;143(Suppl 5):e400S–19S.

57. Jones DR, Detterbeck FC, Morris DE. Tracheal cancers. In: Detterbeck FC, Rivera MP, Socinski MA, et al, editors. Diagnosis and treatment of lung cancer: an evidence-based guide for the practicing clinician. Philadelphia: W. B. Saunders; 2001. p. 408–15.

58. Escalon J, Detterbeck F. Carcinoid tumors. In: Shields T, LoCicero JI, Reed C, et al, editors. General thoracic surgery. 7th edition. Philadelphia: Lippincott Williams & Wilkins; 2009. p. 1539–54.

59. Mineo TC, Guggino G, Mineo D, et al. Relevance of lymph node micrometastases in radically resected endobronchial carcinoid tumors. Ann Thorac Surg 2005;80(2):428–32.

60. Schrevens L, Lorent N, Dooms C, et al. The role of PET scan in diagnosis, staging, and management of non-small cell lung cancer. Oncologist 2004; 9(6):633–43.

61. Stamatis G, Freitag L, Greschuchna D. Limited and radical resection for tracheal and bronchopulmonary carcinoid tumour: report on 227 cases. Eur J Cardiothorac Surg 1990;4:527–33.

62. Filosso PL, Rena O, Donati G, et al. Bronchial carcinoid tumors: surgical management and long-term outcome. J Thorac Cardiovasc Surg 2002;123(2): 303–9.

63. Chughtai T, Morin J, Sheiner N, et al. Bronchial carcinoid–twenty years' experience defines a selective surgical approach. Surgery 1997;122: 801–8.

64. Mezzetti M, Raveglia F, Panigalli T, et al. Assessment of outcomes in typical and atypical carcinoids according to latest WHO classification. Ann Thorac Surg 2003;76(6):1838–42.

65. Nicholson SA, Ryan MR. A review of cytologic findings in neuroendocrine carcinomas including carcinoid tumors with histologic correlation. Cancer 2000;90(3):148–61.

66. Okike N, Bernatz PE, Woolner LB. Carcinoid tumors of the lung. Ann Thorac Surg 1976;22(3): 270–7.

67. Silvestri GA, Gonzalez AV, Jantz M, et al. Methods of staging for non-small cell lung cancer: diagnosis and management of lung cancer, 3rd ed: American College of Chest Physicians evidence-based clinical practice guidelines. Chest 2013;143(Suppl 5): e211S–50S.

68. Rivera M, Mehta AC, Wahidi MM. Establishing the diagnosis of lung cancer: diagnosis and management of lung cancer, 3rd ed: American College of Chest Physicians evidence-based clinical practice guidelines. Chest 2013;143(Suppl 5):e142S–65S.

69. Detterbeck FC, Rivera MP. Clinical presentation and diagnosis. In: Detterbeck FC, Rivera MP, Socinski MA, et al, editors. Diagnosis and treatment

of lung cancer: an evidence-based guide for the practicing clinician. Philadelphia: W.B. Saunders; 2001. p. 45–72.

70. Iyoda A, Hiroshima K, Nakatani Y, et al. Pulmonary large cell neuroendocrine carcinoma: its place in the spectrum of pulmonary carcinoma. Ann Thorac Surg 2007;84(2):702–7.

71. Younossian A, Brundler M, Totsch M. Feasibility of the new WHO classification of pulmonary neuroendocrine tumors. Swiss Med Wkly 2002;132:535–40.

72. den Bakker MA, Willemsen S, Grünberg K, et al. Small cell carcinoma of the lung and large cell neuroendocrine carcinoma interobserver variability. Histopathology 2010;56(3):356–63.

Ectopic Cushing and Other Paraneoplastic Syndromes in Thoracic Neuroendocrine Tumors

Diego Ferone, MD, PhD*, Manuela Albertelli, MD, PhD

KEYWORDS

- Cushing • Corticotropin • Cortisol • Neuroendocrine tumors • Paraneoplastic syndrome

KEY POINTS

- Overproduction of corticotropin by the pituitary gland or extrapituitary tumors leads to hypercortisolism or Cushing syndrome.
- Diagnosis of suspected Cushing syndrome involves 3 major steps: confirmation of hypercortisolism, differentiation between corticotropin-independent and corticotropin dependent causes of Cushing syndrome, and distinction between pituitary and ectopic corticotropin production.
- When ectopic corticotropin is produced by malignancies, circulating corticotropin and cortisol levels are extremely high, the duration of symptoms is shorter, and the clinical phenotype is atypical compared with pituitary-dependent Cushing disease.
- A definitive diagnosis of ectopic corticotropin secretion should require stringent criteria, including reversal of the clinical picture after resection of the tumor and/or demonstration of corticotropin immunohistochemical staining within the tumor tissue.
- Various neoplasms can produce corticotropin, especially those originating from neuroendocrine cells.
- After small cell lung carcinoma (SCLC) and carcinoid tumors, the subsequent most commonly reported tumors causing ectopic corticotropin secretion are harbored in the thymus (11%) and pancreas (8%).
- The main conclusion that can be drawn from the most recently published series is that more than half of the tumors producing ectopic corticotropin secretion were found in the lung or in the thymus, whereas, including MTC and pheocromocytomas, two-thirds were in the thorax, neck, or adrenal glands.
- As in Cushing disease, major symptoms and signs include central obesity, primary or secondary amenorrhea in female patients, hirsutism, acne, violaceous skin striae, easy bruising, hypertension, glucose metabolism imbalance, fatigue, muscle weakness, mental changes or emotional disturbances, hyperpigmentation, and acanthosis nigricans.
- Due to the difficulties in differentiating the source of ectopic corticotropin and although the ectopic tumor represents the minority of all cases of Cushing syndrome, an accurate biochemical as well as radiological work-up is strongly recommended.

Continued

The authors have nothing to disclose.
Endocrinology Unit, Department of Internal Medicine and Medical Specialties, Center of Excellence for Biomedical Research, IRCCS AOU San Martino-IST, University of Genoa, viale Benedetto XV, Genoa 16132, Italy
* Corresponding author.
E-mail address: ferone@unige.it

Continued

- Surgery represents first-line treatment in these patients; however, differently from pituitary corticotropin-dependent Cushing, these cases are generally responsive to somatostatin analog therapy, at least in terms of clinical and biochemical control of the paraneoplastic syndrome.
- Hyponatremia is a common feature in patients with lung cancer.
- Ectopic acromegaly is rare, and since the discovery of growth hormone (GH)–releasing hormone (GHRH) approximately 30 years ago, only 74 cases have been reported in the literature.
- Carcinoid syndrome is a rare feature in bronchial carcinoid patients.
- Another rare cause of endocrine syndrome associated with carcinoid tumor is malignant hypercalcemia and includes ectopic production of parathormone (PTH) or PTH-related peptide (PTH-rp) by the tumor.

ECTOPIC CUSHING SYNDROME

Overproduction of corticotropin by the pituitary gland or extrapituitary tumors leads to hypercortisolism or Cushing syndrome.[1,2] Definition and recognition of the 2 forms of corticotropin-dependent Cushing syndrome is a challenging task. Although a majority of these cases are diagnosed as Cushing disease secondary to an corticotropin-secreting pituitary adenoma, 10% to 15% of them may result in the ectopic corticotropin and/or corticotropin-releasing hormone (CRH) overproduction, which is mainly caused by lung or, more rarely, gastroenteropancreatic or other neuroendocrine tumors.[1,3] Cushing syndrome is associated with major morbidity, especially metabolic and cardiovascular complications, osteoporosis, psychiatric changes, and cognitive impairment. Moreover, exacerbation of prior autoimmune diseases is also seen and all of these systemic complications lead to quality-of-life impairment and increased mortality, regardless of the oncologic outcome of the affected patients.

A diagnosis of suspected Cushing syndrome involves 3 major steps: confirmation of hypercortisolism, differentiation between corticotropin independent and corticotropin-dependent causes of Cushing syndrome, and distinction between pituitary and ectopic corticotropin production.[4] Because normalization of cortisol hypersecretion by the selective removal of a pituitary adenoma or of a solitary bronchial carcinoid tumor has a high probability of resolving the condition, it is essential to distinguish ectopic corticotropin secretion from the more common Cushing disease and, in the former, to make every effort to localize the source of ectopic corticotropin production.[4]

Various benign and malignant tumors have been found associated with ectopic corticotropin secretion. In most cases, when ectopic corticotropin is produced by malignancies, circulating corticotropin and cortisol levels are extremely high, the duration of symptoms is shorter, and the clinical phenotype is atypical compared with pituitary-dependent Cushing disease. Conversely, ectopic corticotropin secretion is often associated with several neuroendocrine tumors with different aggressiveness and which produce the typical signs and symptoms of Cushing syndrome, with a biochemical resemblance to pituitary Cushing disease.[4]

For this reason, it has been stated that a definitive diagnosis of ectopic corticotropin secretion should require stringent criteria, including reversal of the clinical picture after resection of the tumor and/or demonstration of corticotropin immunohistochemical staining within the tumor tissue. Unfortunately, however, these criteria are not applicable to several of the reported cases of ectopic corticotropin secretion.[4] Primary lesion resection cannot be curative in disseminated tumors nor can lack of immunostaining in a biopsy specimen disprove ectopic corticotropin secretion, because only a subpopulation of tumor cells within the tumor mass may actually secrete corticotropin.

Various neoplasms can produce corticotropin, especially those originating from neuroendocrine cells. Initially, these tumors have been recognized based on the characteristics of the neoplastic cells, APUD cells.[4] Small cell lung carcinoma (SCLC); carcinoid tumors, especially of the lungs, thymus, and gastrointestinal tract; islet cell cancers; pheochromocytomas; and medullary thyroid carcinomas (MTCs) are the most frequent along with several miscellaneous tumors, including paraganglioma, neuroblastoma, prostate, breast, kidney, stomach, ovary, melanoma, colon, leukemia, and anorectal cancer, which all have been associated with ectopic Cushing syndrome.[4] In the past, SCLCs accounted for most cases of ectopic corticotropin secretion.[4] In recent surveys, however, the preponderance of these tumors has been substantially reduced in favor of other histologic types.[4] Analysis reveals that the lung is still the most likely organ to harbor an ectopic source of corticotropin, being the origin of more than 45% of tumors: most cases are bronchial carcinoids (>25%) followed by SCLCs and adenocarcinomas (approximately 20%). In the most recent series, for the first time, the frequency of bronchial carcinoids resulted as higher than that of SCLCs, demonstrating the change in referral patterns. When SCLCs were excluded from the analysis, the bronchial carcinoid frequency was as high as 32% of all cases of ectopic corticotropin secretion.

The next most commonly reported tumors causing ectopic corticotropin secretion are harbored in the thymus (11%) and pancreas (8%). Other sources are mostly related to tumors with neuroendocrine differentiation, such as MTCs (6%) and adrenal pheochromocytomas (5%). Only 6% to 8% of histologically confirmed cases derived from nonendocrine, nonpulmonary tumors. These cancers comprise ovarian carcinomas (>2%), anorectal carcinomas (2%), neuroblastoma (1%), uterine cervix carcinomas, prostate cancers, and a few other rare tumors.

The main conclusion that can be drawn from the most recently published series is that more than half of the tumors producing ectopic corticotropin secretion were found in the lung or in the thymus, whereas, including MTC and pheocromocytomas, two-thirds were in the thorax, neck, or adrenal glands.[5,6] Only one-third of primary tumors have been found in the abdomen, most frequently in the pancreas (8%) or the colon (4%).

As in Cushing disease, major symptoms and signs include central obesity, primary or secondary amenorrhea in female patients, hirsutism, acne, violaceous skin striae, easy bruising, hypertension, glucose metabolism imbalance, fatigue, muscle weakness, mental changes or emotional disturbances, hyperpigmentation, and acanthosis nigricans (**Table 1**).

Due to the difficulties in differentiating the source of ectopic corticotropin and although the ectopic source represents the minority of all cases of Cushing syndrome, an accurate biochemical work-up is strongly recommended.[7] High-dose dexamethasone (DEX) can be used to discriminate ectopic corticotropin syndrome from the more common classic Cushing disease. A suppression of more than 50% of the basal cortisol (and corticotropin) levels can be observed in more than 80% of patients with Cushing disease.[7] Conversely, in general, ectopic corticotropin is insensitive to exogenous glucocorticoid administration. Because the diagnostic utility of high-dose DEX test can

Table 1 Clinical symptoms and signs of Cushing syndrome	
Obesity	Hyperglycemia
Violaceous skin striae	Hyperlipemia
Hypertension	Hypercalciuria
Fatigue or weakness	Polyuria
Muscle weakness	Polydipsia
Easy bruising	Increased thrombotic risk
Mental change or emotional lability	Hypogonadism
Hyperpigmentation	Osteoporosis
Acanthosis nigricans	Fungal infection
Primary or secondary amenorrhea in female patients	Acne and hirsutism

be limited, however, when available, inferior petrosal sinuses sampling (IPSS) with measurement of CRH-stimulated corticotropin is strongly recommended.[7] Moreover, because adenomas can be incidentally discovered in up to 10% of the normal population, IPSS is advised for patients with corticotropin-dependent Cushing syndrome and concomitant presence of a pituitary adenoma smaller than 6 mm, particularly when biochemical suppressive and/or stimulating tests display conflicting results.[7] IPSS can demonstrate the ratio of the corticotropin level in the central sinuses relative to the peripheral samples. A central/peripheral ratio of 2 before the administration of CRH and a ratio of higher than 3 after its administration strongly suggest Cushing disease.[7] Although a positive result is highly suggestive of Cushing disease, however, false-negative results might be more common than previously estimated (2%–4%). In cases of a negative response, clinicians should perform a careful search for an ectopic source of corticotropin.[7]

Because the most likely site of ectopic corticotropin-producing tumors is thorax and these tumors are frequently bronchial carcinoids, accurate radiologic search is mandatory. Localization of these tumors can also, however, be challenging. These lesions are mostly small, as well as slow growing, and conventional imaging studies, such as CT and MRI scans, identify the tumor in only 50% of cases.[7] The primary tumor can remain occult long after a diagnosis of Cushing.[7] Functional imaging studies, such as fludeoxyglucose F 18 (FDG) positron emission tomography (PET), and somatostatin receptor scrintigraphy (SRS), are complementary imaging tools to detect carcinoids.[7] SRS might be superior to FDG PET in detecting bronchial carcinoids. FDG PET can distinguish highly active proliferative tumors, whereas bronchial carcinoids usually have a low proliferation index and are slow growing small lesions.[7] The success of SRS in localizing tumors depends, however, on the presence of somatostatin receptors, which have been identified on many cells of neuroendocrine origin,[7] as well as from the tumor size. Therefore, single-photon emission CT reconstruction of the planar images is strongly recommended. The radiolabeled somatostatin, analog, octreotide, can bind with high affinity to somatostatin receptor subtypes 2 and 5.[7] Bronchial carcinoids generally express both receptor subtypes. Nevertheless, these tumors may show heterogeneity in the degree of somatostatin receptor expression or may be very small, under the detection limit of this technique.[7] The diagnostic sensitivity of SRS is approximately 25% to 73% for the detection of an ectopic source of corticotropin secretion.[7] Ilias and colleagues[5] reported that the sensitivity of SRS is approximately 49%, and it is insufficient for lesions that are not displayed by CT scan or MRI. Zemskova reported 57% sensitivity and a 79% positive predictive value for SRS for detecting ectopic corticotropin-producing tumors.[8] The use of a single imaging tool may not be sufficient to diagnose ectopic corticotropin-secreting tumors. Therefore, conventional and functional imaging studies should be used in combination when needed.[7] More recently, gallium-68 somatostatin receptor PET and PET/CT have become new and valuable diagnostic tools for patients with neuroendocrine tumors. These highly accurate techniques should be considered first-line diagnostic imaging methods in patients with suspicious thoracic and/or gastroenteropancreatic neuroendocrine tumors because they combine the advantages of PET technology with the use of radiotracers able to identify somatostatin receptor–positive tumors with higher sensitivity and specificity, even for even lesions smaller than 10 mm.[9] **Fig. 1** shows an ideal algorithm for diagnosis of Cushing syndrome due to ectopic corticotropin production.

Surgery represents first-line treatment in patients with ectopic Cushing syndrome; however, differently from pituitary corticotropin-dependent Cushing, cases with ectopic tumors are generally responsive to somatostatin analogs therapy, at least in terms of clinical and biochemical control of the paraneoplastic syndrome. Additional more aggressive treatments are used in cases resistant

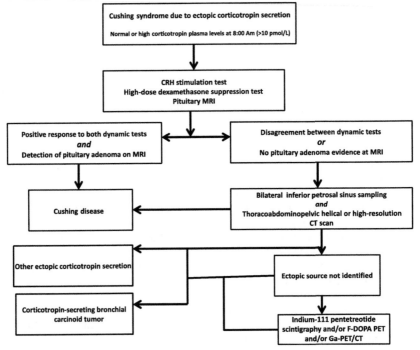

Fig. 1. Diagnostic algorithm in Cushing syndrome caused by ectopic corticotropin secretion. F-DOPA PET, fluoro-dihydroxyphenylalanine positron emission tomography; Ga-PET, Gallium-DOTA positron emission tomography.

to biotherapy. Fewer data are available on the so-called targeted therapies (everolimus, sunitinib, and so forth) compared with neuroendocrine tumors of different origin; however, the initial report and data derived from large series, including thoracic neuroendocrine tumors, are promising for lung and thymic carcinoids as well.[10] Among chemotherapies, only temozolomide, alone or combined with capecitabine, has shown significant results, although in small series.[3]

SYNDROME OF INAPPROPRIATE ANTIDIURETIC HORMONE SECRETION

Hyponatremia is common feature in patients with lung cancer.[11] As a recent retrospective analysis demonstrated, the syndrome of inappropriate antidiuretic hormone (SIADH) secretion, as a hallmark of SCLC, can be found in approximately 10% to 15% of them but only in 2% to 4% of all non–SCLC patients.[11] In SCLC patients, SIADH is diagnosed predominantly in advanced stages and may induce a significant reduction in plasma sodium levels. Clinical symptoms, such as dizziness, tremor, agitation, and other neuropsychiatric disorders, have to be taken into consideration for the diagnosis of clinically relevant hyponatremia. Mild symptoms, such as fatigue, occur in mild (plasma sodium = 130–134 mmol/L) and in moderate (plasma sodium = 125–129 mmol/L) hyponatremia.[3] Clinical symptoms can aggravate in hyponatremia (plasma sodium <125 mmol/L). SIADH is a common finding in SCLC patients with euvolemic hyponatremia.[11] SCLC belongs to a class of the most malignant solid tumors. At the time of diagnosis, most of the patients (90%) are classified as patients with limited, palliative treatment options. Due to the advanced age of this cohort (median 70 years), comorbidities, such as cardiovascular diseases or respiratory insufficiency, influence the therapeutic strategies. Short treatment periods with tolvaptan (15 mg/d) resulted in sufficiently stabilizing sodium levels in a majority of the cases. Correction of sodium and amelioration of clinical symptoms may help to improve the prognosis in patients with advanced disease. In addition, hyponatremia management may shorten inpatient treatment periods and minimize emergency room calls. Furthermore, treatment with tolvaptan is a recommendable and safe treatment option for terminally ill patients requiring emergency treatment in a palliative situation (**Box 1**, **Table 2**).[12]

ECTOPIC ACROMEGALY

Ectopic acromegaly is rare, and since the discovery of growth hormone (GH)–releasing hormone

---

Box 1
Symptoms and signs of syndrome of inappropriate antidiuretic hormone secretion

Mild to moderate

Headache, lethargy, slowness, poor concentration, depressed mood, lack of attention, impaired memory, nausea, restlessness, instability of gait and falls, muscle cramps, tremor

Advanced

Confusion, disorientation, somnolence, vomiting, hallucinations, acute psychosis, limb weakness, dysarthria

Severe

Seizures, hemiplegia, severe somnolence, respiratory insufficiency, coma, death

---

(GHRH) approximately 30 years ago, only 74 cases have been reported in the literature. The values for GHRH, which are usually undetectable in pituitary acromegaly, are elevated in patients with acromegaly due to ectopic tumor, reaching values hundreds- or thousands-fold above normal values. Laboratory results, including basal and post–oral glucose GH values, serum insulin-like growth factor 1, and plasma GHRH should be evaluated. GHRH assay is available, however, in few, but experienced, laboratories around the

---

Table 2
Diagnosis of syndrome of inappropriate antidiuretic hormone secretion

Primary diagnostic features	
Plasma osmolality	<275 mOsm/kg
Urine osmolality	>100 mOsm/kg
Euvolemia or hypervolemia	—
Urinary sodium	>30 mmol/L
Normal thyroid, kidney, and adrenal function	—
No diuretic drugs	—

Secondary diagnostic features
  Uric acid less than 4 mg/dL
  BUN less than 10 mg/dL
  FE (Na) greater than 1%; FE (urea) greater than 55%
  Failure to improve hyponatremia after 0.9% physiologic solution infusion
  Improvement of hyponatremia after water restriction	

Abbreviations: BUN, blood urea nitrogen; FE, fractional excretion.

world. Clinically, unique and unexpected features in acromegalic patients, including respiratory wheezing or dyspnea, facial flushing, peptic ulcers, and renal stones, are sometimes helpful in alerting physicians diagnosing nonpituitary endocrine tumors. Pituitary gland may be normal or enlarged at MRI, which may be difficult to interpret, especially in multiple endocrine neoplasia type 1 (MEN 1) patients, where the association of a microprolactinoma (more rarely a clinically nonfunctioning pituitary adenoma) to a pancreatic tumor secreting GHRH may be misleading. When reliable, plasmatic GHRH shows an excellent specificity for the diagnosis, using a threshold of 250 to 300 ng/L, and is an appropriate tool for following up patients during treatments. These tumors may have a good overall prognosis, even in metastatic setting, which represent 50% of cases. Surgical approach is recommended and, when a complete tumor resection is feasible, results, in most patients, in long-lasting remission. In such cases, GHRH concentration normalizes and its increase is an accurate indicator of tumor recurrence. In noncured patients, somatostatin analogs not only control pituitary GH secretion but also may inhibit abnormal ectopic GHRH production. MEN 1 mutation should be systematically investigated in patients with a pancreatic tumor.[12,13]

CARCINOID SYNDROME

Carcinoid syndrome is a rare feature in bronchial carcinoid patients. A review of the literature suggests a variable range of 2% to 7% of thoracic neuroendocrine tumors displaying carcinoid syndrome in various series. This is usually associated with recurrent carcinoid tumor in the presence of hepatic metastasis. Bronchial carcinoids in some cases are not able to sustain the clinical syndrome because (1) pulmonary tissue may contain large amounts of monoamine oxidase that inhibits the serotonin; (2) the functional potential capacity of pulmonary carcinoids is less compared with gastroenteric carcinoids, and they are detected earlier and removed before they reach the size able to produce a significant amount of serotonin; and (3) metastasis to the liver produces the syndrome because the liver is not able to metabolize the large amounts of serotonin produced. Although there are a few reports of cases of the carcinoid syndrome in bronchial carcinoid, they were usually present before the excision of the primary tumor. The presence of carcinoid syndrome after successful surgical excision of primary tumor without any evidence of abdominal disease is usually suggestive of nodal recurrence.[14] Recurrent bronchial neuroendocrine tumors presenting with carcinoid syndrome also may occur many years after curative surgery in the absence of abdominal disease.[15] Apart from surgery, somatostatin analogs are effective in controlling symptoms and reducing biochemical markers of the disease. Depending on the grading, other medical approaches may be considered for those patients resistant to somatostatin analogs.

HYPERPARATHYROIDISM LINKED TO ECTOPIC PARATHORMONE AND PARATHORMONE-RELATED PEPTIDE PRODUCTION

Another rare cause of endocrine syndrome associated with carcinoid tumor is malignant hypercalcemia and includes ectopic production of PTH or PTH-rp by the tumor, extensive lytic bone metastases, primary hyperparathyroidism, tumor-associated PGEs, interleukin-1β (previously known as osteoclast-activating factor), transforming growth factor β, and receptor activator of nuclear factor κβ ligand. Transforming growth factor β1 regulates the messenger ribonucleic acid stability of PTH-rp. The hypercalcemia of malignancy seen in lymphosarcoma and anal sac apocrine gland adenocarcinoma is commonly caused by tumor-associated PTH-rp. PTH-rp is a 16-kDa protein with significant sequence identity to PTH, suggesting that the hypercalcemia seen in PTH-rp–associated malignancy is due to the ability of PTH-rp to act and function like PTH. In addition to malignant hypecalcemia, other forms of hypercalcemia should be distinguished first. Among these, laboratory pitfalls (presence of lipemia and sample hemolysis), acute renal failure, hypervitaminosis D, hypoadrenocorticism, granulomatous disease, and others, may be considered. Removal of the tumor produces, in a majority of cases, a normalization of calcium levels in cases of absence of a metastatic disease. PTHrP-secreting tumors should be considered in the differential diagnosis of patients with neuroendocrine tumors who present with hypercalcaemia and a disproportionately low PTH. PTHrP tumors may be underestimated because the assay is difficult to perform and may not be requested. In hypercalcemic patients, the standard management acutely includes intravenous fluids administration, diuretics, and intravenous bisphosphonate.

REFERENCES

1. Hashemzadeh S, Asvadi Kermani A, Ali-Asgharzadeh A, et al. Ectopic Cushing's syndrome secondary to pulmonary carcinoid tumor. Ann Thorac Surg 2013;95:1797–9.

2. Phan AT, Öberg K, Choi J, et al, North American Neuroendocrine Tumor Society (NANETS). NANETS consensus guideline for the diagnosis and management of neuroendocrine tumors: well-differentiated neuroendocrine tumors of the thorax (includes lung and thymus). Pancreas 2010;39:784–98.

3. Öberg K, Hellman P, Ferolla P, et al, ESMO Guidelines Working Group. Neuroendocrine bronchial and thymic tumors: ESMO Clinical Practice Guidelines for diagnosis, treatment and follow-up. Ann Oncol 2012;23(Suppl 7):vii120–3.

4. Isidori AM, Lenzi A. Ectopic ACTH syndrome. Arq Bras Endocrinol Metabol 2007;51:1217–25.

5. Ilias I, Torpy DJ, Pacak K, et al. Cushing's syndrome due to ectopic corticotropin secretion: twenty years' experience at the National Institutes of Health. J Clin Endocrinol Metab 2005;90:4955–62.

6. Isidori AM, Kaltsas GA, Pozza C, et al. The ectopic adrenocorticotropin syndrome: clinical features, diagnosis, management, and long-term follow-up. J Clin Endocrinol Metab 2006;91:371–7.

7. Anaforoğlu I, Ersoy K, Aşık M, et al. Diagnosis of an ectopic adrenocorticotropic hormonesecreting bronchial carcinoid by somatostatin receptor scintigraphy. Clinics (Sao Paulo) 2012;67:973–5.

8. Zemskova MS, Gundabolu B, Sinaii N, et al. Utility of various functional and anatomic imaging modalities for detection of ectopic adrenocorticotropin-secreting tumors. J Clin Endocrinol Metab 2010;95:1207–19.

9. Treglia G, Castaldi P, Rindi G, et al. Diagnostic performance of Gallium-68 somatostatin receptor PET and PET/CT in patients with thoracic and gastroenteropancreatic neuroendocrine tumors: a meta-analysis. Endocrine 2012;42:80–7.

10. Pavel ME, Hainsworth JD, Baudin E, et al, RADIANT-2 Study Group. Everolimus plus octreotide long-acting repeatable for the treatment of advanced neuroendocrine tumours associated with carcinoid syndrome (RADIANT-2): a randomised, placebo-controlled, phase 3 study. Lancet 2011;10(378): 2005–12.

11. Petereit C, Zaba O, Teber I, et al. A rapid and efficient way to manage hyponatremia in patients with SIADH and small cell lung cancer: treatment with tolvaptan. BMC Pulm Med 2013;13:55.

12. Gross P. Clinical management of SIADH. Ther Adv Endocrinol Metab 2012;3:61–73.

13. Borson-Chazot F, Garby L, Raverot G, et al, GTE Group. Acromegaly induced by ectopic secretion of GHRH: a review 30 years after GHRH discovery. Ann Endocrinol (Paris) 2012;73:497–502.

14. Gola M, Doga M, Bonadonna S, et al. Neuroendocrine tumors secreting growth hormone-releasing hormone: pathophysiological and clinical aspects. Pituitary 2006;9:221–9.

15. Ganti S, Milton R, Davidson L, et al. Facial flushing due to recurrent bronchial carcinoid. Ann Thorac Surg 2007;83:1196–7.

Functional Imaging Evaluation in the Detection, Diagnosis, and Histologic Differentiation of Pulmonary Neuroendocrine Tumors

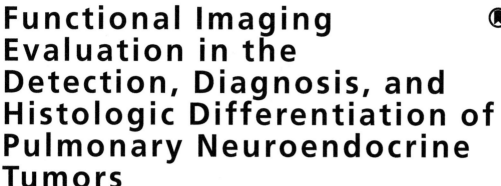

Filippo Lococo, MD[a],*, Giorgio Treglia, MD[b],
Alfredo Cesario, MD[c], Massimiliano Paci, MD[a],
Angelina Filice, MD[d], Annibale Versari, MD[d],
Pier Luigi Filosso, MD[e]

KEYWORDS

- Pulmonary neuroendocrine tumors • pNETs • PET-CT scans • Radiometabolic evaluation

KEY POINTS

- Distinct features of different pulmonary neuroendocrine tumors (pNETs) include their pathologic characteristics as well as their clinical behavior, epidemiology, treatment, and prognosis.
- Typical carcinoids (TCs) are indolent neoplasms with a good prognosis, whereas atypical carcinoids (ACs) have a less indolent behavior with a certain propensity for metastatic spread. Both are well-differentiated pulmonary NETs are optimally treated with complete surgical excision.
- More aggressive pNETs, such as large cell neuroendocrine lung cancer and small cell lung cancer, often present with local invasion, thoracic lymph nodal metastases, and distant spread. As a result, affected patients may not be candidates for surgical resection and are treated with chemotherapy with or without radiation therapy, showing a poor prognosis.
- Taking into account the different biologic behavior of various pNET subtypes, achieving an accurate preoperative diagnosis is a key element for planning the best strategy of care.
- Recent evidence suggests that, even when surgery is indicated, the extent of both pulmonary resection and lymph nodal dissection are determined by the cytohistologic characteristics of pNETs.
- TCs and ACs share structural radiological findings and a clear differentiation is not possible through radiological findings only. The functional imaging evaluation using nuclear medicine techniques has improved in the last two decades with the aim of helping the physicians in the challenging clinical decision-making process of these rare entities.

Continued

The authors have nothing to disclose.

[a] Unit of Thoracic Surgery, Department of Nuclear Medicine, IRCCS-Arcispedale Santa Maria Nuova, viale risorgimento 80, Reggio Emilia 42121, Italy; [b] Department of Nuclear Medicine, Oncology Institute of Southern Switzerland, Bellinzona 6500, Switzerland; [c] Scientific Direction, IRCCS-San Raffaele Pisana, Via della Pisana, 235, Rome 00163, Italy; [d] Department of Nuclear Medicine, IRCCS-Arcispedale Santa Maria Nuova, viale risorgimento 80, Reggio Emilia 42121, Italy; [e] Department of Thoracic Surgery, University of Torino, via Giuseppe Verdi 8, Torino 10124, Italy

* Corresponding author.

E-mail address: filippo_lococo@yahoo.it

Thorac Surg Clin 24 (2014) 285–292

http://dx.doi.org/10.1016/j.thorsurg.2014.04.004

Continued

- Because a certain or definitive diagnosis may not be easily obtained, radiometabolic evaluation represents a sort of noninvasive biopsy trying to correlate as accurately as possible the uptake pattern of pNETs (using different tracers) with the histologic types. Positron emission tomography (PET), using different tracers, has potential in the work-up process of pNETs. It may detect functional abnormalities even before the tumors become morphologically evident on conventional imaging.
- Not relying on dimensional criteria, PET is more accurate than conventional imaging for the disease extent assessment, restaging, and therapy response. Tracer uptake at PET imaging may be evaluated visually or by using semiquantitative measures such as the maximal standardized uptake value.
- The development of integrated PET-CT scans, has greatly contributed to a more accurate delineation of areas of increased tracer uptake, overcoming the limits of patients repositioning when the two images were acquired independently and fused afterward. Several PET tracers have been proposed for the evaluation of pNETs. The potential role of functional imaging evaluation using fluorine-18 fluorodeoxyglucose and somatostatin analogues labeled with gallium-68 in well-differentiated pNETs (TCs and ACs) with particular attention on clinical and surgical implications should be considered.

INTRODUCTION

It is well known that the distinct features among the different pulmonary neuroendocrine tumors (pNETs) include their pathologic characteristics as well as their clinical behavior, epidemiology, treatment, and prognosis. In addition, typical carcinoids (TCs) are indolent neoplasms with a good prognosis, whereas atypical carcinoids (ACs) have a less indolent behavior with a certain propensity for metastatic spread. Both these well-differentiated pNETs are optimally treated with complete surgical excision. Conversely, more aggressive pNETs, such as large cell neuroendocrine lung cancer (LCNEC) and small cell lung cancer (SCLC), often present with local invasion, thoracic lymph nodal metastases, and distant spread. Affected patients may not be candidates for surgical resection and are treated with chemotherapy with or without radiation therapy, showing a poor prognosis.[1,2]

Taking into account the different biologic behavior of various pNETs subtypes, the achievement of an accurate preoperative diagnosis is a key element for planning the best strategy of care in such patients.

Recent evidence suggests that even when surgery is indicated, the extent of both pulmonary resection and lymph nodal dissection are determined by the cytohistologic characteristics of pNETs.[2,3]

Unfortunately, TCs and ACs share structural radiological findings and a clear differentiation between these pNETs is not possible through radiological findings only.[4,5]

The functional imaging evaluation using nuclear medicine techniques has improved in the last two decades,[6] aiding physicians in the challenging clinical decision-making process for such rare entities. Because a certain or definitive diagnosis may not be easily obtained, the radiometabolic evaluation would represent a sort of noninvasive biopsy, which tries to correlate the uptake pattern of NETs (using different tracers) with the histologic types as accurately as possible.

Positron emission tomography (PET), using different tracers, has potential in the work-up process of pNETs. It may detect functional abnormalities even before the tumors become morphologically evident on conventional imaging. Moreover, not relying on dimensional criteria, PET is more accurate than conventional imaging for the disease extent assessment, restaging, and therapy response. Tracer uptake by PET imaging may be evaluated visually or by using semiquantitative measures such as the maximal standardized uptake value (SUVmax). Finally, the development of integrated PET-CT scans has greatly contributed to a more accurate delineation of areas of increased tracer uptake, overcoming the limits of patient repositioning when the two images were acquired independently and fused afterward.

Several PET tracers have been proposed for the evaluation of pNETs. This article, however, focuses on the potential role of functional imaging evaluation using fluorine-18 fluorodeoxyglucose (^{18}F FDG) and somatostatin analogues labeled with gallium-68 (^{68}Ga) DOTA-peptides in well-differentiated pNETs (TCs and ACs) with particular attention on clinical and surgical implications.

ROLE OF THE ^{18}F FDG–PET-CT SCAN

Because ^{18}F FDG is a glucose analogue, this tracer may be very useful in detecting malignant lesions that usually present high glucose metabolism.[7] Tumors that are slow growing (ie, carcinoid tumors) exhibit a lower glucose uptake compared with other aggressive malignancies (ie, LCNECs and SCLCs).[8]

As a result, LCNECs and SCLC[9] show higher ^{18}F FDG uptake compared with bronchial carcinoids (BCs) that were often reported as tumors that are not ^{18}F FDG-avid.[9] This understanding led many physicians to consider this technique as a tool of limited value for the diagnosis of BCs (low sensitivity and a limited role in the diagnostic work-up). This conviction originated from the first work on ^{18}F FDG-PET in BCs by Erasmus and colleagues,[10] in 1998, who reported a series of seven cases of pulmonary carcinoids of which three were visually negative on ^{18}F FDG-PET (all TCs), three were hypometabolic (2 TCs and 1 AC) and, thus, they were erroneously categorized as benign nodules. Only one case (TC) revealed a visual positivity and SUVmax of 6.6. Subsequent studies (**Table 1**), however, did not confirm these findings. In fact, both TCs and ACs may show a variable FDG uptake according to tumor proliferation. Wartski and colleagues[11] described two carcinoids with intense ^{18}F FDG uptake (SUVmax 4.8 and 10.6) and, later, Kruger and colleagues[12] reported 13 pulmonary carcinoids of which 54% were hypermetabolic ^{18}F FDG-PET.

Daniels and colleagues[13] studied 16 subjects and found a sensitivity value of 75% for ^{18}F FDG-PET in carcinoids detection. Chong and colleagues[9] found that the uptake in 6 of 7 carcinoids (86%) was higher than the standard threshold value (>2.5). Kayani and colleagues[14] reported that 9 of 13 patients with BCs (69%) showed significant ^{18}F FDG uptake and were considered to have malignant lesions. Jindal and colleagues[15] found an overall detection rate of 70% by ^{18}F FDG-PET in a series of 20 carcinoids. It is interesting that the method of assessment of the nodule uptake is pivotal for an adequate evaluation of the accuracy of ^{18}F PET for BCs. In fact, as recently reported by Stefani and colleagues,[16] the sensitivity of ^{18}F PET for carcinoids was generally investigated based on a visual assessment of a SUVmax cutoff. Regarding the visual assessment, the PET scan results were typically interpreted as positive when the nodule activity was greater than the background mediastinal pool activity.[9,10]

Table 1
Literature overview: [18]F FDG-PET scan in the evaluation of pulmonary carcinoids

Author, Year	Number of Subjects	Histology	Detection Rate (%)
Wartski et al,[11] 2004	2	1 TC, 1 AC	100
Kruger et al,[12] 2006	15	12 TCs, 1 AC	54
Daniels et al,[13] 2007	16	11 TCs, 5 ATs	75
Chong et al,[9] 2007	7	2TCs, 5 ACs	86
Kayani et al,[14] 2009	13	11 TCs, 2 ACs	69
Jindal et al,[15] 2011	20	13 TCs, 7 ACs	70
Stefani et al,[16] 2013	25	24 TCs, 1 AC	48 (positive result if SUVmax >2.5) 96 (positive result if SUVmax >1.5)

When the SUVmax was used to define the PET positivity, a cut-off of 2.5 (derived from the first experiences with the use of ^{18}F FDG-PET in lung carcinoma) was commonly applied.[13,14] BCs, especially TCs, show a lower metabolic activity with respect to lung carcinoma; therefore, a different SUVmax cut-off should be applied for the evaluation of ^{18}F FDG uptake. In light of these considerations, the cut-off value of 2.5 no longer seems adequate, especially for TCs. In fact, if a cut-off of 1.5 was fixed, no false-negative results would have been present in the series by Erasmus and colleagues[10] (0 of 6 subjects) and Kayani and colleagues[14] (0 of 11 subjects) and reduced false-negative rates of 23% would have been found in the series by Jindal and colleagues.[15] [18]F FDG uptake of BCs was related to the histologic type and proliferation rate. Indeed, it is generally known that neoplasms that are slow growing exhibit a lower glucose uptake compared with other aggressive malignancies. Applying these assumptions to BC metabolism, as well as the ^{18}F FDG-PET imaging, it may be assumed that PET sensitivity is poor when considering typical forms only, whereas it may be comparable to PET sensitivity in non-small cell lung cancer (NSCLC) cases when ACs are taken into account. Robust data support the assumption that ACs present with a significantly higher ^{18}F FDG uptake than TCs because of their more aggressive behavior and high proliferation rate.[9,11–15] A recent retrospective study[17] confirmed that ACs have higher ^{18}F FDG uptake and showed that a SUVmax greater than or equal to 6 had a predictive value of greater than 95% for malignant histology (AC vs TC). For lung carcinomas it is well known that the intensity of the ^{18}F FDG uptake can be directly correlated to the tumor dimensions.[18] Erasmus and colleagues[10] and Kruger and colleagues[19] demonstrated that the SUVmax was directly related to tumor diameter for BCs. In addition, Daniels and colleagues[12] reported a correlation between the ^{18}F FDG uptake and the size of the neoplasm, even if SUVmax values were not calculated. Finally, the SUVmax values were reported to be related to patient survival in poor-differentiated pNETs (LCNECs and SCLCs).[19,20] Even though similar findings have been observed in well-differentiated pNETs (TCs and ACs),[9,12,17] the prognostic value of ^{18}F FDG-PET scan in such tumors must be defined and further studies on large cohorts are needed.

In conclusion, ^{18}F FDG-PET sensitivity is suboptimal when identifying overall pulmonary carcinoid tumors. Indeed, although significant uptake values are generally observed in ACs (comparable with those observed in NSCLC cases), TCs are associated with a very low uptake and ^{18}F FDG-PET imaging sensitivity is remarkably reduced in these tumors. Nevertheless, when a BC is strongly suspected by clinical or radiological findings, even a very low ^{18}F FDG uptake should not be considered as a negative result.[16] In these cases, a surgical resection or, at least, a noninvasive biopsy, should be mandatory.

ROLE OF [68]GA DOTA-PEPTIDES PET-CT SCAN

Somatostatin is a peptide hormone that regulates the endocrine system and controls neurotransmission and cell proliferation via the interaction with G-protein–coupled somatostatin receptors (SSTRs) as well as inhibiting the release of several hormones. High SSTR density may be found on many endocrine-related tumors cells, including pNETs. The density of these receptors is related to the degree of tumor differentiation, the most well-differentiated ones (ie, TCs) expressing the highest density. Recent development of novel tracers (ie, ^{68}Ga DOTA-peptides) has allowed imaging of SSTRs by PET. In detail, ^{68}Ga DOTA-peptides bind to SSTRs over-expressed on NET cells. [68]Ga

DOTA-peptide structure includes an active part, which binds to SSTR (DOTA0-Phe1-Tyr3-octreotide [DOTA-TOC], DOTA0-Tyr3-octreotide [DOTA-NOC], and DOTA-Tyr3-octreotate [DOTA_TATE]), a chelant (DOTA), and a positron-emitting isotope (^{68}Ga). The most relevant differences between these compounds are their variable affinities to SSTR subtypes[21]: all can bind to SSTR2 and SSTR5, only DOTANOC also has a good affinity for SSTR3. However, the observed differences in receptor binding affinities has not yet found a direct clinical correlation; therefore, there is no indication that such differences might be related to specific advantages in clinical use.[6] From a practical point of view, ^{68}Ga DOTA-peptides present several advantages, including an easy labeling and synthesis process.[22] The uptake does not depend on cell metabolism (compared with 2-fluoro-5-hydroxy-L-tyrosine [^{18}F DOPA] or ^{18}F FDG) and noninvasively provides information on SSTR expression with direct therapeutic implications. Finally, the ^{68}Ga DOTA-peptides PET with integrated CT fusion has superior resolution and anatomic localization, offering higher advantages compared with the traditional indium-111 (^{111}In) pentetreotide receptor scintigraphy for diagnosis and therapeutic planning.[14] [68]Ga DOTA-peptides PET or PET-CT usefulness has been initially reported in well-differentiated abdominal NETs.[23,24] Various studies have demonstrated advantages in various NET (including BCs) preoperative workups (**Table 2**).[14,15,23,25,26,28,29] However, the rarity of BCs strongly limits the acquisition of large and robust evidences on their clinical use. In addition, ^{68}Ga DOTA-peptides use is still limited to specialized centers.[6] Hofmann and colleagues[25] evaluated eight subjects with histologically proven metastatic carcinoid tumors by SSTR scintigraphy and ^{68}Ga DOTATOC–PET-CT (6 abdominal and 2 bronchial). [68]Ga DOTATOC-PET was able to identify all lesions in eight subjects, whereas SSTR scintigraphy detected 85% of those previously detected by the traditional radiological imaging.

Koukouraki and colleagues[26] reported ^{68}Ga DOTATOC-PET overall sensitivity of 90.47% in 15 carcinoid tumors of various sites scheduled for yttrium-90 (^{90}Y) DOTATOC therapy. Among these, two pulmonary carcinoids presented with eight neoplastic localizations and ^{68}Ga DOTATOC–PET-CT was able to identify seven out of eight. Gabriel and colleagues[30] evaluated 84 cases of NETs (5 BCs) using ^{68}Ga DOTATOC–PET-CT. The investigators reported higher sensitivity for tumor detection by ^{68}Ga DOTATOC–PET-CT compared with single-photon emission computed tomography (SPECT) or CT. The overall ^{68}Ga DOTATOC–PET-CT scan sensitivity was 97%, specificity 92%, and accuracy 96%. Ambrosini and

Table 2
Literature overview: ^{68}Ga DOTA-peptides PET scan in the evaluation of pulmonary carcinoids

Author, Year	Number of Subjects	Histology	Detection Rate (%)
Hofman et al,[25] 2001	2[a]	N/A	100
Koukouraki et al,[26] 2006	2[a]	N/A	100[b]
Kumar et al,[27] 2009	3	3 TCs	100
Ambrosini et al,[28] 2009	11	N/A	82
Kayani et al,[14] 2009	13[c]	11 TCs, 2 ACs	100
Jindal et al,[15] 2011	20	13 TCs, 7 ACs	95
Venkitaraman et al,[29] 2014	26	21 TCs, 5 ACs	96

Abbreviation: N/A, not applicable.
[a] Metastatic carcinoid tumors of the lung.
[b] Among 8 metastatic lesions, the detection rate was 87.5% (7 of 8 lesions).
[c] Both primary and recurrent or metastatic pulmonary carcinoids were included.

colleagues[28] evaluated 11 subjects with pulmonary carcinoids with no false-positive findings on ^{68}Ga DOTATOC–PET-CT scan (detection rate of 82%). They also detected a higher number of lesions with this tool, compared with traditional CT scan (37 vs 21, respectively).

Because TCs have been reported to express higher SSTRs than do ACs, it seems logical that TCs may show higher radiotracer uptake on SSTR-based imaging studies.[15] Finally, some ^{68}Ga DOTA-peptides PET false-negative results in pNETs may be due to low expressing of SSTRs tumors. Conversely, inflammatory diseases can yield false-positive results with ^{68}Ga DOTA-peptides PET because SSTRs are also overexpressed by inflammatory cells.[25,31,32] In conclusion, despite the preliminary encouraging results with the ^{68}Ga DOTA-peptides PET scan efficacy in detection of well-differentiated pNETs, further analysis should be carried out to definitively assess the role of this interesting diagnostic method.

DUAL-TRACER PET EVALUATION USING ^{68}GA DOTA-PEPTIDES AND ^{18}F FDG

The solitary pulmonary nodule (SPN) evaluation a major challenge for clinicians. Several imaging modalities and algorithms to detect and predict the likelihood of malignancy have been used. SPNs (especially the round nodules) are difficult to accurately diagnose based purely on the limited sensitivity of noninvasive imaging. This is due to the common technical biopsy limits (especially in small-size and centrally located lesions) and the high frequency of benign lesions detected during radiological assessment. In this setting, functional imaging can assist the physicians with this challenging process, providing valuable information for SPN diagnosis and differentiation. The ^{18}F FDG–PET-CT can be helpful in distinguishing benign from malignant lesions; however, when a BC is suspected, low or absent lesion metabolic activity does not completely exclude a malignancy. On the other hand, in case of increased ^{18}F FDG uptake, the suspicion of BC enters into the differential diagnosis with other entities, including some rare lung neoplasms and/or NSCLCs with atypical radiological features. Otherwise, ^{68}Ga DOTA-peptides are more specific tracers in the detection of pulmonary carcinoids: a positivity at ^{68}Ga DOTA-peptides PET is highly predictive for a definitive pulmonary carcinoid diagnosis. Nevertheless, the ^{68}Ga DOTA-peptides uptake lack does not exclude the diagnosis of pulmonary carcinoid, especially when differentiation is poor. In light of these considerations, the scientific community[33] has started to investigate the possibility of using both functional techniques with a combined dual-tracer (^{68}Ga DOTA-peptides PET-CT and ^{18}F FDG) PET-CT evaluation in case of suspected neuroendocrine tumors. Few reports on the use of ^{68}Ga DOTA-peptides in comparison with ^{18}F FDG have been published.[14,15,29,32] Kumar and colleagues[27] evaluated the role of a combination of ^{18}F FDG–PET-CT scan and ^{68}Ga DOTA-peptides PET-CT scan in differentiating seven cases of bronchial masses, including three BCs: two TCs and one AC. They found that TCs had slight ^{18}F FDG and high ^{68}Ga DOTATOC uptake. In contrast, ACs presented with moderate ^{18}F FDG and high ^{68}Ga DOTATOC uptake. The investigators recommended the combined use of ^{18}F FDG and ^{68}Ga DOTA-peptides PET-CT scans in patients with bronchial tumors in large clinical series settings. A retrospective study by Kayani and colleagues[14] compared ^{68}Ga DOTA-peptides and ^{18}F FDG–PET-CT in 18 pNETs, including 13 BCs. The investigators reported a good correlation between tumor differentiation and ^{68}Ga DOTA-TATE uptakes. Indeed, TCs showed significantly higher ^{68}Ga DOTA-peptides and lower ^{18}F FDG uptake compared with high-grade pNETs. On the other hand, variable uptake was documented with ^{18}F FDG. Nearly half of the cases showed no uptake, whereas only a few patients presented a low one. Moreover, no false-positive ^{68}Ga DOTATATE uptake was observed, but three false-positive ^{18}F FDG uptakes due to tissue inflammation were seen. Overall, the 68Ga DOTA-TATE superiority for the well-differentiated pNETs assessment was evident. Jindal and colleagues[15] studied 20 subjects with pulmonary carcinoids (13 TCs, 7 ACs) with ^{18}F FDG and ^{68}Ga DOTATOC scans, confirming a higher ^{68}Ga DOTATOC uptake in TCs and an increased ^{18}F FDG uptake in ACs. Furthermore, the ^{68}Ga DOTATOC SUVmax uptake was significantly higher in TCs than in ACs ($P<.001$). The investigators concluded that the combination of both PET tracers may be useful in the histopathologic pNET subtype prediction.

Finally, Venkitaraman and colleagues[29] performed the first prospective study on ^{68}Ga DOTATOC and ^{18}F FDG comparison in 32 subjects with suspicion of clinical BC. The overall ^{68}Ga DOTATOC–PET-CT sensitivity, specificity, and accuracy were 96.15%, 100%, and 96.87%, respectively; whereas those of ^{18}F FDG–PET-CT were 78.26%, 11.1%, and 59.37%, respectively. The ^{68}Ga DOTATOC–PET-CT sensitivity was superior in patients with TCs (100% vs 80%), whereas ^{18}F FDG–PET-CT sensitivity was higher in ACs (100% vs 61.9%).

Based on medical literature data, the most frequent TCs uptake pattern at dual-tracer PET-CT imaging is a high radiolabeled somatostatin analogue and low or absent ^{18}F FDG analogue. Conversely, ACs usually present increased ^{18}F FDG uptake and low or moderate radiolabeled somatostatin analogues (**Figs. 1 and 2**).

Moreover, ^{68}Ga somatostatin analogues seem to be the PET tracers of choice in the initial evaluation of patients with clinical suspicion of BCs. In this setting, ^{68}Ga somatostatin analogue PET-CT could be performed initially and, if negative, ^{18}F FDG–PET-CT could be performed.

In conclusion, the combination of ^{68}Ga somatostatin analogue and ^{18}F FDG–PET-CT seems to be helpful in predicting histology when a BC is suspected, making possible a tailored therapeutic approach in these patients.[34] More large prospective studies are needed to validate this diagnostic strategy. Nevertheless, this approach is expensive and its introduction into clinical practice is yet to be realized.

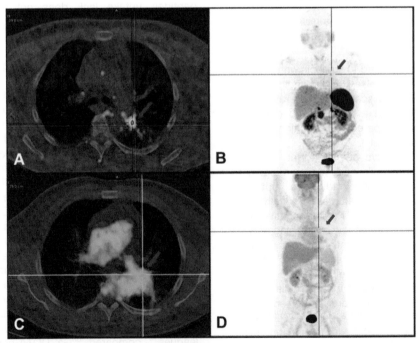

Fig. 1. Metabolic pattern for TC, in CT (*A, C*) and in PET scans (*B, D*). Increased uptake of radiolabeled somatostatin analogues (*A, B*) and low or absent uptake of ^{18}F FDG (*C, D*). *Red arrows* indicate the lesion. (*Courtesy of* IRCCS, Arcispedale, Santa Maria Nuova, Reggio, Emilia, Italy.)

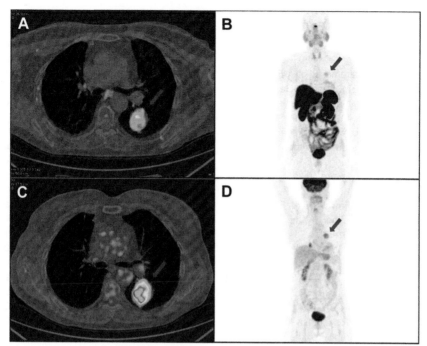

Fig. 2. Functional pattern for AC. Increased uptake (*A, B*) and moderate or low uptake of radiolabeled somatostatin analogues (*C, D*) as studied by CT on the left and by ^{18}F FDG-PET on the right side. *Red arrows* indicate the lesion. (*Courtesy of* IRCCS, Arcispedale, Santa Maria Nuova, Reggio, Emilia, Italy.)

Other Tracers in PC Evaluation

Other PET tracers over ^{18}F FDG and ^{68}Ga somatostatin analogues can be used in the BCs assessment, including carbon-11-hydroxytryptophan and ^{18}F DOPA. Nonetheless, clinical reports are few and results are still controversial.[35–37]

REFERENCES

1. Benson RE, Rosado-de-Christenson ML, Martínez-Jiménez S, et al. Spectrum of pulmonary neuroendocrine proliferations and neoplasms. Radiographics 2013;33:1631–49.
2. Okoye CC, Jablons DM, Jahan TM, et al. Divergent management strategies for typical versus atypical carcinoid tumors of the thoracic cavity. Am J Clin Oncol 2013. http://dx.doi.org/10.1097/COC.0b013e31827a7f6d.
3. Johnson R, Trocha S, McLawhorn M, et al. Histology, not lymph node involvement, predicts long-term survival in bronchopulmonary carcinoids. Am Surg 2011;77:1669–74.
4. de Guevara AC, Burigana F, Nicolini A, et al. Neuroendocrine tumors of the lung: hystological classification, diagnosis, traditional and new therapeutic approaches. Curr Med Chem 2014;21:1107–16.
5. Rindi G, Klersy C, Inzani F, et al. Grading the neuroendocrine tumors of the lung: an evidence-based proposal. Endocr Relat Cancer 2013;21:1–16.
6. Ambrosini V, Nicolini S, Caroli P, et al. PET/CT imaging in different types of lung cancer: an overview. Eur J Radiol 2012;81:988–1001.
7. Vansteenkiste J, Fischer BM, Dooms C, et al. Positron emission tomography in prognostic and therapeutic assessment of lung cancer: systematic review. Lancet Oncol 2004;5:531–40.
8. Higashi K, Ueda Y, Ayabe K, et al. FDG PET in the evaluation of the aggressiveness of pulmonary adenocarcinoma: correlation with histopathological features. Nucl Med Commun 2000;21:707–14.
9. Chong S, Lee KS, Kim BT, et al. Integrated PET/CT of pulmonary neuroendocrine tumors: diagnostic and prognostic implications. AJR Am J Roentgenol 2007;188:1223–31.
10. Erasmus JJ, McAdams HP, Patz EF, et al. Evaluation of primary pulmonary carcinoid tumors using FDG PET. AJR Am J Roentgenol 1998;170:1369–73.
11. Wartski M, Alberini JL, Leroy-Ladurie F, et al. Typical and atypical bronchopulmonary carcinoid tumors on FDG-PET/CT imaging. Clin Nucl Med 2004;29:752–3.
12. Kruger K, Buck AK, Blumstein NM, et al. Use of integrated FDG-PET/CT imaging in pulmonary carcinoid tumors. J Intern Med 2006;260:545–50.
13. Daniels CE, Lowe VJ, Aubry MC, et al. The utility of fluorodeoxyglucose positron emission tomography in the evaluation of carcinoid tumors presenting as pulmonary nodules. Chest 2007;131:255–60.

14. Kayani I, Conry BG, Groves AM, et al. A comparison of 68Ga-DOTATATE and 18 F-FDG PET/CT in pulmonary neuroendocrine tumors. J Nucl Med 2009;50:1927–32.

15. Jindal T, Kumar A, Venkitaraman B, et al. Evaluation of the role of [18 F]FDG-PET/CT and [68Ga]DOTATOC-PET/CT in differentiating typical and atypical pulmonary carcinoids. Cancer Imaging 2011;11:70–5.

16. Stefani A, Franceschetto A, Nesci J, et al. Integrated FDG-PET/CT imaging is useful in the approach to carcinoid tumors of the lung. J Cardiothorac Surg 2013;8:223. http://dx.doi.org/10.1186/1749-8090-8-223.

17. Moore W, Freiberg E, Bishawi M, et al. FDG-PET imaging in patients with pulmonary carcinoid tumor. Clin Nucl Med 2013;38:501–5.

18. Cerfolio RJ, Bryant AS, Ohja B, et al. The maximum standardized uptake values on positron emission tomography of a non-small cell lung cancer predict stage, recurrence and survival. J Thorac Cardiovasc Surg 2005;130:151–9.

19. Blum R, MacManus MP, Rischin D, et al. Impact of positron emission tomography on the management of patients with small-cell lung cancer: preliminary experience. Am J Clin Oncol 2004;27:16471.

20. Pandit N, Gonen M, Krug L, et al. Prognostic value of [18F]FDG-PET imaging in small cell lung cancer. Eur J Nucl Med Mol Imaging 2003;30:7884.

21. Antunes P, Ginj M, Zhang H, et al. Are radiogallium-labelled DOTA-conjugated somatostatin analogues superior to those labelled with other radiometals? Eur J Nucl Med Mol Imaging 2007;34:982–93.

22. Zhernosekov KP, Filosofov DV, Baum RP, et al. Processing of generator produced 68Ga for medical application. J Nucl Med 2007;48:1741–8.

23. Kumar R, Sharma P, Garg P, et al. Role of (68)Ga-DOTATOC PET-CT in the diagnosis and staging of pancreatic neuroendocrine tumors. Eur Radiol 2011;21:2408–16.

24. Prasad V, Ambrosini V, Hommann M, et al. Detection of unknown primary neuroendocrine tumours (CUP-NET) using (68)Ga-DOTANOC receptor PET/CT. Eur J Nucl Med Mol Imaging 2010;37:67–77.

25. Hofmann M, Maecke H, Borner R, et al. Biokinetics and imaging with the somatostatin receptor PET radioligand (68)Ga-DOTATOC: preliminary data. Eur J Nucl Med 2001;28:1751–7.

26. Koukouraki S, Strauss LG, Georgoulias V, et al. Comparison of the pharmacokinetics of 68Ga-DOTATOC and [18F]FDG in patients with metastatic neuroendocrine tumours scheduled for 90YDOTA-TOC therapy. Eur J Nucl Med Mol Imaging 2006;

33:1115–22. http://dx.doi.org/10.1007/s00259-006-0110-x.

27. Kumar A, Jindal T, Dutta R, et al. Functional imaging in differentiating bronchial masses: an initial experience with a combination of (18)F-FDG PET-CT scan and (68)Ga DOTA-TOC PET-CT scan. Ann Nucl Med 2009;23(8):745–51. http://dx.doi.org/10.1007/s12149-009-0302-0.

28. Ambrosini V, Castellucci P, Rubello D, et al. 68Ga-DOTA-NOC: a new PET tracer for evaluating patients with bronchial carcinoid. Nucl Med Commun 2009;30:281–6.

29. Venkitaraman B, Karunanithi S, Kumar A, et al. Role of 68Ga-DOTATOC PET/CT in initial evaluation of patients with suspected bronchopulmonary carcinoid. Eur J Nucl Med Mol Imaging 2014;41:856–64. http://dx.doi.org/10.1007/s00259-013-2659-5.

30. Gabriel M, Decristoforo C, Kendler D, et al. 68Ga-DOTA-Tyr3-octreotide PET in neuroendocrine tumours: comparison with somatostatin receptor scintigraphy and CT. J Nucl Med 2007;48:50818. http://dx.doi.org/10.2967/jnumed.106.035667.

31. Treglia G, Castaldi P, Rindi G, et al. Diagnostic performance of Gallium-68 somatostatin receptor PET and PET/CT in patients with thoracic and gastroenteropancreatic neuroendocrine tumours: a meta-analysis. Endocrine 2012;42:80–7.

32. Vanhagen PM, Krenning EP, Reubi JC, et al. Somatostatin analogue scintigraphy in granulomatous diseases. Eur J Nucl Med 1994;21:497–502.

33. Paci V, Lococo F, Rapicetta C, et al. Synchronous bilateral bronchial carcinoid diagnosed with combined dual tracer (18F-FDG and 68Ga-DOTATOC) PET/CT scans. Rev Esp Med Nucl Imagen Mol 2013. http://dx.doi.org/10.1016/j.remn.2013.08.007.

34. Treglia G, Giovanella L, Lococo F. Evolving role of PET/CTwith different tracers in the evaluation of pulmonary neuroendocrine tumours. Eur J Nucl Med Mol Imaging 2014;41:853–5. http://dx.doi.org/10.1007/s00259-014-2695-9.

35. Treglia G, Lococo F, Petrone G, et al. Pulmonary neuroendocrine tumor incidentally detected by 18F-CH PET/CT. Clin Nucl Med 2013;38:e196–9.

36. Wahlberg J, Ekman B. Atypical or typical adrenocorticotropic hormone-producing pulmonary carcinoids and the usefulness of 11C-5-hydroxytryptophan positron emission tomography: two case reports. J Med Case Rep 2013;7:80.

37. Rufini V, Treglia G, Montravers F, et al. Diagnostic accuracy of [18F]DOPA PET and PET/CT in patients with neuroendocrine tumors: a meta-analysis. Clin Transl Imaging 2013;1:111–22.

The Significance of Histology
Typical and Atypical Bronchial Carcinoids

Mariano García-Yuste, MD, PhD[a],*,
José María Matilla, MD, PhD[b]

KEYWORDS

- Carcinoid tumors • Histology • Surgical procedure • Metastases • SSTR tumor receptors

KEY POINTS

- In carcinoid tumors, histologic classification and stage establishment provide an adequate tumor biologic behavior understanding.
- When nodal affectation is detected, a preoperative histologic confirmation by biopsy is mandatory.
- The progress applied to the diagnosis and treatment of the listed developments demands the knowledge of the number of patients who are surgically treated for this type of tumor per year.

The aim of this article is to answer different questions related to the treatment and prognosis of the bronchial carcinoids, considering the significance of their histology.

Carcinoid tumors are malignant and rare neoplasms that account approximately for 2% to 3% of all primary lung cancers. The distinction between typical and atypical carcinoid was first described by Engelbreth-Holm in 1944[1]; the histologic criteria of this distinction was later established by Arrigoni[2] in 1972. The initial classification of these tumors established in 1982 by the World Health Organization (WHO)[3] has been modified several times. As consequence of clinical and prognostic controversies, new histologic criteria proposed by Travis to separate typical and atypical carcinoids[4] have been considered and accepted by the WHO and International Association for the Study of Lung Cancer (IASLC) 1999 classification of lung tumors.[5]

Taking into account these facts, in the spectrum of the neuroendocrine carcinomas, the gradual deterioration of histologic pattern organization in typical and atypical carcinoid has a significant relationship with their prognosis. In contrast with typical carcinoid (TC), atypical carcinoid (AC) has been defined as a tumor with neuroendocrine morphology and mitotic counts of 2 or more and less than 10 per 2 mm^2 of viable tumor (10 high-power fields, HPF), or the presence of punctate foci of coagulative necrosis.[4] Large areas of geographic necrosis typical of high-grade neuroendocrine carcinomas are not seen.[6] Additionally, descriptions of phenotypic, molecular, and genetic abnormalities were added to these criteria[7] in 2004.

TC has a less aggressive behavior; it rarely relapses after complete surgical resection, and nodal involvement and distant metastases are rare. AC represents, in the spectrum of neuroendocrine lung tumors, an intermediate stage between TC and large and small cell neuroendocrine carcinomas. Surgery is the mainstay of treatment; nevertheless, the main prognostic factors in these neoplasms are not precisely defined in the literature.

The experience gained through multicenter research could allow a more adequate study and satisfactory answers to several questions.

SPANISH MULTICENTER EXPERIENCE

From 1980 to 2009, the authors expanded their experience in 927 surgically treated bronchial carcinoids. Among them, 796 patients had a TC, and

[a] University Hospital of Valladolid, Valladolid University, Avd. Ramón y Cajal N° 3, 47005 Valladolid, Spain;
[b] University Hospital of Valladolid, Avd. Ramón y Cajal N° 3, 47005 Valladolid, Spain
* Corresponding author.
E-mail address: mgyuste2@hotmail.com

Thorac Surg Clin 24 (2014) 293–297
http://dx.doi.org/10.1016/j.thorsurg.2014.05.003

127 patients had an AC. At the beginning, these patients were retrospectively collected, and from 1999, the rest of patients were studied prospectively. A lymph nodal dissection was systematically performed in the prospective group. All patients affected by carcinoid were pathologically coded according to the 2009 tumor, nodal, metastases (TNM) lung cancer staging standards. All histologic samples were reviewed to be classified by the WHO classification, including Travis's criteria for AC (**Table 1**).

Surgical procedures performed in both TC and AC are described in **Fig. 1**.

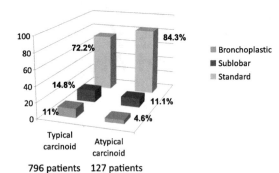

Fig. 1. Surgical procedures performed in both TC and AC.

WHAT IS THE NODAL INVOLVEMENT IMPACT IN THESE TUMORS?

In lung cancer, tumor size and lymph node involvement are local anatomic factors that strongly influence prognosis. Their classification in different degrees and the establishment of stages provide an adequate understanding of the behavior of the tumor as well as the opportunities to treat them.

Bronchial carcinoid staging demonstrates that the number of patients in stage I gradually decreases from TC to AC.[8] On the other hand, the number of stage II and III patients notably increases in AC.[8] This fact indirectly reflects the importance of histologic aggressiveness as a determining factor in tumor size and nodal involvement (**Fig. 2**).

As in other primary lung cancers, in carcinoid tumors lymph node involvement is a primary prognostic factor that is dependent on the histologic tumor type. The analysis of this prognostic factor in a large number of TC and AC cases confirms this element (**Fig. 3**).

On the other hand, in patients analyzed by the Spanish Multicentre Study of Neuroendocrine Lung Tumors, differences among patients with AC were noted in this retrospective and prospective analysis (performing sampling [retrospective group] or mediastinal nodal dissection [prospective group] in all patients). An important increase in lymph nodal involvement was detected in prospective group patients in both TC and AC (**Fig. 4**); additionally the proportion of N2/N1 involvement in the prospective group was significantly higher than that found in the

retrospective group.[8] Nevertheless, there have been few studies that have analyzed in depth the reasons for the impact of the presence of lymph node involvement in the prognosis of bronchial carcinoids.

The frequency of recurrences after surgery is different between TC and AC. In TC, 22 of 796 patients (2.76%) developed metastases, and 10 patients had local recurrence, including 3 cases associated with distant metastases. In AC, 27 of 127 patients (21.26%) had distant metastases, of which 5 cases were associated with local recurrence. Additionally, 4 patients presented with isolated local recurrence.

Most patients with TC who developed metastasis or local recurrence were in stage I, and more than 55% were alive after treatment. Among AC patients, 66% had lymph node metastases, and 80% of them died after treatment because of their recurrence. The analysis of these results enables the authors to confirm that nodal invasion did not demonstrate an obvious influence in the prognosis of TC, while it did in AC.

The knowledge of the histologic limits of TC and AC established by the new WHO classification contributes, without a doubt, to the realization of a better valuation of the proportional significance that nodal involvement and histologic grade have in the prognosis of both groups of tumors.

The role of positron emission tomography (PET) imaging is not yet well defined in bronchial carcinoids, with widely disparate sensitivity.[9] When AC lymph nodal involvement is detected by PET/computed tomography (CT), single-photon

Table 1						
Spanish multicenter experience						
n. Cases	Global 923	%	Retrospective 1980–1998 389	%	Prospective 1999–2009 534	%
Typical carcinoid	796	86.2	345	88.7	451	84.5
Atypical carcinoid	127	13.8	44	11.3	83	15.5

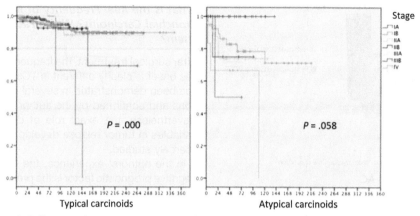

Fig. 2. Prognostic influence of stage status in TC and AC. Univariate analysis (Kaplan-Meier).

emission CT (SPECT) Indium In 111pentetreotide, or Ga-DOTA-TOC PET/CT,[10,11] a preoperative histologic confirmation by endobronchial ultrasound (EBUS)/endoscopic ultrasound (EUS) or video mediastinoscopy is mandatory to determine the suitability of a neoadjuvant treatment.

WHEN IS A CONSERVATIVE RESECTION OF PARENCHYMA IN CARCINOID TUMORS WORTHWHILE?

A conservative bronchoplastic lung resection could be considered in different modalities in centrally located TC and AC, avoiding pneumonectomy.

Nevertheless, Detterbeck noted that the bronchoplastic resection incidence might vary according to the different centers' experience (reported sleeve resection rates between 2% and 14%).[12]

Most central cN0 carcinoids are TCs. The available data suggest that a lung-sparing operation is equivalent to a larger resection, at least in TC patients. Satisfactory long-term survival after sleeve resection in TC has, in fact, been demonstrated.

Considering these facts, the question is when a parenchyma-sparing resection is appropriate. The authors agree with Detterbeck, that in centrally located TC, the use of lung-sparing bronchoplastic techniques could influence local recurrence in some cases. This observation needs an intraoperative adequate surgical margin-free pathologic confirmation by frozen section.

Peripheral TCs have been occasionally resected by wedge or segmental resections. However, today it is generally accepted that the best results in terms of long-term survival are achieved with a lobectomy. In patients with limited pulmonary function, a standard segmentectomy achieves better results compared with a broad wedge resection. The increase risk of local recurrence in a peripheral AC treated with a sublobar resection makes it, in the authors' opinion, not advisable. Consequently, lobectomy is also the standard of care for peripheral AC (**Table 2**).

To summarize, the choice of surgical procedure in carcinoid tumors should be determined by the histologic characteristics and the ascertainment

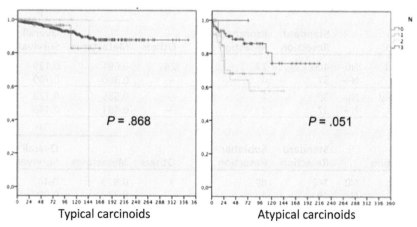

Fig. 3. Prognostic influence of N-status in TC and AC. Univariate analysis (Kaplan Meier).

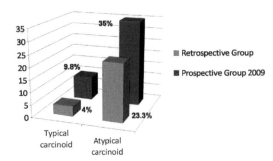

Prospective Group: systematic nodal mediastinal dissection

Fig. 4. N+ in TC and AC.

of tumor local spread during surgery. Both in TC and AC, and independent of their central or peripheral location, systematic hilar and mediastinal lymph nodal dissection should always carried out. Concerning lung parenchyma-sparing resections, in a sleeve lobectomy for a centrally located TC, an intraoperative adequate surgical margin pathologic verification is mandatory. In peripheral AC, the increased risk of local recurrence after a limited resection makes it not advisable.

Tumor Local Recurrence and Distant Metastasis Treatment and Prognosis

Local and distant recurrences are not very frequent in bronchial carcinoids, and their treatment has not been sufficiently yet clarified. There are, in fact, few clinical experiences on this issue. Answering several questions concerning the frequency, the diagnosis, the treatment and the prognosis of the local and distant tumor recurrence in TC and AC is therefore essential.

What Is the Real Frequency of Recurrence in Bronchial Carcinoids? Which Factors Influence Them?

After surgical treatment, the frequency of metastases onset is clearly different in TCs and ACs. This has been demonstrated in several recent publications and confirmed by the authors' experience.[8] Nevertheless, the exact role of different clinical variables in tumor relapse development has been scarcely studied.

In the authors' experience, the only significant negative prognostic factor is the presence of lymph nodal metastases in ACs.

How Should the Follow-Up Designed?

In general, the bronchial carcinoid follow-up should be organized according to the primary lung cancer's general rules.

The free-of-disease interval and survival after recurrence of carcinoids are long but different in TCs and ACs.

Somatostatin scintigraphy may be useful in diagnosis of recurrences, but the current validity of these results should be established.

By this means, it is necessary to carry out exploration of the primary tumor before the surgical treatment and/or determine receptors of somatostatin analogues by means of immunohistochemistry. Nevertheless, somatostatin scintigraphy is expensive and available in selected centers, only. Furthermore, tumors that do not express somatostatin receptors (SSTR) receptors (30% of carcinoids) should be excluded.

Fluorodeoxyglucose (^{18}FDG)-PET scan is usually not sensible in bronchial carcinoids, due to their

Table 2
Influence of surgical procedure and nodal involvement in the presence of metastases; overall survival and local recurrence was analyzed considering central versus peripheral location

Central Location		Standard Resection	Bronchoplastic Resection	Others	Metastases	Overall Survival	Local Recurrence
Typical carcinoid	N0	400	77	24	0.691	0.129	0.004
	N+	37	4	—	0.386	0.709	0.202
Atypical carcinoid	N0	39	2	—	0.585	0.723	—
	N+	27	3	—	0.481	0.145	0.893

Peripheral Location		Standard Resection	Sublobar Resection	Others	Metastases	Overall Survival	Local Recurrence
Typical carcinoid	N0	142	89	3	0.975	0.447	0.375
	N+	19	1	—	0.773	0.900	0.950
Atypical carcinoid	N0	30	13	—	0.45	0.599	0.018
	N+	11	2	—	0.763	0.727	0.345

low biologic uptake; Ga-DOTA-TOC PET/CT or SPECT-CT–Indium In 111 pentetreotide is contrariwise much more valuable, but very expensive.

How to Treat Metastases?

Three factors should guide treatment of recurrences: location, metastases spread, and the patient's general conditions. Surgery, chemotherapy/radiotherapy, biotherapy (somatostatin analogues and alpha interferon) and symptomatic treatment are the available means.

In patients with liver metastases and poor general conditions, loco-regional treatments (embolization, chemoembolization, radiofrequency, and cryosurgery) have been suggested.[13] In patients without extrahepatic disease and fulfilling the Milano criteria, liver transplantation guarantees an acceptable mean and median survival.[14]

Could We Consider as Useful the Design of New Diagnosis and Treatment Strategies in Carcinoid Pulmonary Tumors?

The effect on neuroendocrine pulmonary tumors of the recently developed SSTR analogues, which constitute specific subtypes of somatostatin, has proved to be advantageous for the control of the cell spread in these tumors.[15]

With an aim to precise the significance of the presence of SSTR receptors in these tumors, spanish multicenter study of neuroendocrine lung tumors-spanish society of pneumonology and thoracic surgery (EMETNE-SEPAR) has begun research on histologic samples of carcinoid tumors—preferably atypical—and large-cell neuroendocrine carcinomas. The aim is to specify the diagnosis and therapeutic profitability of the somatostatin analogues in connection with the presence of SSTR in these tumors, through the evaluation of repercussion of the existence of SSTR tumor receptors during the tumor recurrence follow-up, the response to treatment of recurrence, and patient survival.

Under the aforementioned situations, the progress applied to the diagnosis and treatment of the listed developments demands the knowledge of the annual number of patients who are surgically treated for this type of tumor per year. The limitations of the study are given, both by the limited particularization in papers of the number of patients treated per year during a specific period, and by the scarce multicenter studies with enough patients.

REFERENCES

1. Engelbreth-Holm J. Benign bronchial adenomas. Acta Chir Scand 1944;90:383–409.

2. Arrigoni MG, Woolner LB, Bernatz PE. Atypical carcinoid tumor of the lung. Thorac Cardiovasc Surg 1972;64:413–21.

3. The World Health Organization histological typing of lung tumors. Second edition. Am J Clin Pathol 1982; 77:123–36.

4. Travis WD, Rush W, Flieder DB, et al. Survival analysis of 200 pulmonary neuroendocrine tumors with clarification of criteria for atypical carcinoid and its separation from typical carcinoid. Am J Surg Pathol 1998;22:934–44.

5. Travis WD, Sobin LH. Histologic typing of lung and pleural tumours; international histologic classification of tumours (No.1). New York: Springer-Verlag; 1999.

6. Rekhtman N. Neuroendocrine tumors of the lung. An update. Arch Pathol Lab Med 2010;134:1628–38.

7. Vallieres E, Shepherd FA, Crowley J, et al, International Association for the Study of Lung Cancer International Staging Committee and Participating Institutions. The IASLC Lung Cancer Staging Project: proposals regarding the relevance of TNM in the pathologic staging of small cell lung cancer in the forthcoming (seventh) edition of the TNM classification for lung cancer. J Thorac Oncol 2009;4:1049–59.

8. García-Yuste M, Matilla JM, Cueto A, et al, Members of the Spanish Multicenter Study of Neuroendocrine Tumors of the Lung by the Spanish Society of Pneumonology and Thoracic Surgery (EMETNE-SEPAR). Typical and atypical carcinoid: analysis of the experience of the Spanish multicenter study of neuroendocrine tumors of the lung. Eur J Cardiothorac Surg 2007;31:192–7.

9. Erasmus J, McAdams HP, Patz EF Jr, et al. Evaluation of primary pulmonary carcinoid tumors using FDG PET. AJR Am J Roentgenol 1998;170:1369–73.

10. Rodrigues M, Traub-Weidinger T, Li S, et al. Comparison of In-DOTA-DPhe-Tyr-octeotride and In-DOTA-lanreotide scintigraphy and dosimetry in patients with neuroendocrine tumours. Eur J Nucl Med Mol Imaging 2006;33:532–40.

11. Ambrosini V, Castellucci P, Rubello D, et al. 68Ga-DOTA-NOC: a new PET tracer for evaluating patients with bronchial carcinoid. Nucl Med Commun 2009; 30:281–6.

12. Detterbeck FC. Management of carcinoid tumors. Ann Thorac Surg 2010;89:998–1005.

13. Filosso PL, Ruffini E, Oliaro A, et al. Long-term survival of atypical bronchial carcinoids with liver metastases, treated with octreotide. Eur J Cardiothorac Surg 2002;21:913–7.

14. Blonski WC, Reddy KR, Shaked A, et al. Liver transplantation for metastatic neuroendocrine tumor: a case report and review of the literature. World J Gastroenterol 2005;11(48):7676–83.

15. García-Yuste M, Matilla JM, Gonzalez-Aragoneses F. Neuroendocrine lung tumors. Curr Opin Oncol 2008; 20:148–54.

Bronchoplastic Procedures for Carcinoid Tumors

Marco Anile, MD[a], Daniele Diso, MD[a],
Erino A. Rendina, MD[a,1], Federico Venuta, MD[b,*,1]

KEYWORDS

- Carcinoid tumor • Neuroendocrine tumor • Bronchoplastic procedure • Sleeve resection

KEY POINTS

- Carcinoid tumors are relative rare lung neoplasms; they may arise centrally or peripherally.
- For central lesions, bronchoplastic procedures, particularly sleeve resections, are safe.
- Bronchoplastic procedures, particularly sleeve resections, should be the reference for treatment when anatomically and oncologically indicated, independently from pulmonary function for central lesions.

Bronchial carcinoids are rare neuroendocrine tumors: the annual incidence is approximately 2.3 to 2.8 cases per 1 million population.[1] They account for less than 5% of all bronchopulmonary tumors[2] and about 25% of all carcinoids.[2,3] They are classified as typical and atypical; both of them show a different and more favorable prognosis when compared with non–small cell lung cancer, with atypical carcinoids behaving more aggressively. They may present as central and peripheral lesions. The natural history of these tumors is strictly related to the lymph node status.[4,5] Between N0 and N1 patients no statistical significant difference has been observed; however, N2 bronchial carcinoid tumors show a dismal prognosis, also because at this stage they are predominantly atypical. This is the reason why also for these tumors complete lyphadenectomy should be performed.

Approximately 20% of all carcinoid tumors present as pure endobronchial polyp-like lesions without gross radiologically detectable involvement of the bronchial wall and lung parenchyma.[2]

This unusual presentation and their indolent clinical course have contributed to competition in this specific setting between surgical resection and different endoscopic techniques, namely neodymium:yttrium-aluminum-garnet laser, diathermy, and cryosurgery.[6–9] However, carcinoids arising within the bronchus with or without a limited extension through the bronchial wall are clearly suitable for resection with bronchoplasty (bronchial sleeve resection or wedge) when indicated. This can be performed with or without parenchymal resection and offers a definitive solution in such cases.[10] Wedge resection and lobectomy are the procedure of choice when the lesion is within the parenchyma, accordingly to its site and extension; pneumonectomy is extremely rare.

Carcinoid tumors tend to be indolent and complete resection with disease-free margins is mandatory. Broncoplasty procedures look appropriate[11,12] and in these situations they rarely require pulmonary artery reconstruction.[13]

Bronchial sleeve resections are required when a tumor infiltrates the origin of a lobar bronchus but

[a] Department of Thoracic Surgery, University of Rome Sapienza, Rome, Italy; [b] Department of Thoracic Surgery, Policlinico Umberto I, University of Rome Sapienza, V.le del Policlinico 155, Rome 00166, Italy
[1] Fondazione Eleonora Lorillard Spencer Cenci.
* Corresponding author.
E-mail address: Federico.venuta@uniroma1.it

Thorac Surg Clin 24 (2014) 299–303
http://dx.doi.org/10.1016/j.thorsurg.2014.04.003
1547-4127/14/$ – see front matter © 2014 Elsevier Inc. All rights reserved.

not to the extent that pneumonectomy is required. Additionally, these procedures might be indicated when N1 lymph nodes involve the bronchial takeoff; however, this happens rarely with carcinoid tumors. Bronchial sleeve resections have been also described for more peripheral lesions involving the segmental bronchi.[14–16]

There are several aspects peculiar to the carcinoid population of patients; they differentiate this group from those with lung cancer and they may also contribute to simplify the technical details. In fact, Prince-Thomas[17] has performed the first reported bronchial reconstruction in a patient with this type of tumor. These lesions often show a well-defined base of implant allowing less aggressive procedures; even complete parenchyma-sparing bronchial resections may be performed in selected cases.[18,19] On the contrary, lung cancer with such presentation is extremely rare. This approach is indicated when the tumor involves the main bronchus only, allowing clear resection margins without removing any lung tissue. In this setting, also bronchial wall wedge resections have been reported.

A typical presentation of these lesions, when they are centrally located, shows limited extrabronchial spread, a small base of implant, a normal distal bronchial tree, and no lymph node involvement.

The distal lung status is also extremely important. These are slow-growing lesions and the long-lasting local progression may favor chronic infection of the parenchyma. If complete occlusion of the bronchial lumen occurs, laser recanalization should be performed[20] to drain and clean the distal airway, assess quality and function of the lung, evaluate more reliably the distal end of the base of implant of the tumor, and treat infection. A cycle of antibiotics and pulmonary rehabilitation contribute to ameliorate the clinical status before surgery and improves results. In our experience, this approach has been performed in four patients undergoing sleeve resection for carcinoids; in all the other cases there was only partial obstruction of the bronchial lumen allowing drainage of secretions and distal progression of the fiberoptic bronchoscope.

SURGICAL TECHNIQUE

The technical details are identical to those of bronchial sleeve resections performed for lung cancer. Most bronchial sleeve resections can be planned preoperatively. Thus, fiberoptic bronchoscopy should always be performed by the operating surgeon to have a precise idea of the anatomic details. If performed elsewhere, it should be repeated. Histology should be confirmed before surgery. An intercostal pedicle flap should be prepared before entering the chest.[21,22] We routinely use it to wrap the anastomosis. It favors protection and revascularization of the bronchial anastomosis and separates it from the arterial side when a combined bronchovascular reconstruction is performed, avoiding bronchoarterial fistulas. Also, a small dehiscence can be "contained" by the wrapped muscle. Alternatively, the anastomosis can be encircled by thymic or mediastinal tissue.

Most of the bronchial sleeve resections are performed by removing the right and left upper lobes along with a sleeve of main bronchus. Frozen sections should always be performed to confirm complete resection. Radical hilar and mediastinal lymphadenectomy may be easily performed after the lobe has been removed and the bronchial stumps lie open in the operative field. The bronchial anastomosis is performed with interrupted 4/0 PDS sutures. The first two or three sutures are placed on the far end of the cartilaginous ring; they are immediately tied extraluminally by the operator and the first assistant. Interrupted sutures are placed on the remaining cartilaginous ring and the membranous portion and are left untied. On the cartilaginous portion the stitches are usually placed submucosally. Placing the sutures in this order helps prevent caliber discrepancies and torsion of the anastomosis; it is almost never required to intussuscept the distal stump, even in case of evident size discrepancies. The sutures are progressively tied starting from the mediastinal side where the first stitches have been previously closed. The anastomosis should be tension free; this is done by dividing the pulmonary ligament. On the right side, the pericardium can be incised around the inferior pulmonary vein to help upward mobilization of the residual lobes. When only the main bronchus has to be resected (this happens more often on the left side for anatomic reasons) the technique of reimplantation of the distal stump is the same.

Y sleeve resection with reimplantation of the upper lobe may be required in case of tumors arising in the lower bronchus on the left and in the intermediate bronchus on the right, when the lobar carina is involved. A few technical details should be kept in mind in case of Y sleeve resection with reimplantation of the upper lobe bronchus. This bronchus is usually short and minute, especially on the right side; the pulmonary artery and lung parenchyma are extremely close to the bronchus, worsening the exposure on the mediastinal side of the anastomosis. Size discrepancies with the right main bronchus are not rare and in extreme cases the smaller side can be intussuscepted. However, more often, the larger bronchial stump works as a stent, increasing the caliber of the anastomosis and helping to keep the distal part open.

Bronchoplasties at the level of the segmental bronchus are less common. They can be performed especially in pathologic conditions other than lung cancer, including low-grade malignant tumors, metastatic lesions, and strictures caused by tuberculosis. Advantages include less tension on the distal stump, more efficient blood supply to the airway, and placement of the anastomosis inside the lung parenchyma; this allows an outside pull because of negative pressure. In these cases, the fissure should not be entered, the intersegmentary plane should be isolated as for a standard segmentectomy, and the bronchus should be reimplanted with the anastomotic technique previously described. Development of bare surface of the lung after isolating the segment to be removed rarely causes problems during the postoperative course.

COMMENT

Carcinoid tumors often occur in young and fit patients (mean age younger than 50 years; atypical carcinoids show older age).[3] They are low-grade tumors and for N0-N1 lesions long-term prognosis is extremely encouraging. Thus, quality of life is crucial. For this reason parenchymal-sparing procedures should always be considered when planning surgery; they include wedge resections for peripheral tumors and bronchial reconstructions for central lesions. Notwithstanding the clear benefit of this approach, the incidence of sleeve resections in the different series varies with a wide range, from 1.4% to 41% (**Table 1**). This is probably related to the time when the different series were produced (mostly 1980s and 1990s). More recent reports include larger series of patients.[41] Although technically demanding, bronchoplastic procedures are now definitively accepted as valuable options for these patients. Surgery should be carefully planned in advance, preparing the patient for the procedure.

There is only one study[42] comparing bronchoplasty procedures (including sleeve and wedge) between carcinoids and primary lung cancer (18 and 80 patients, respectively). In this report the carcinoid group showed less anastomotic complications; also, nonsurgical complications were less frequent, probably because of the younger age of these patients (38.5 vs 61.5, respectively).

Frozen sections should always be available and confirm clear resection margins. From the different series it is impossible to extrapolate survival after

Table 1 Incidence of bronchial sleeve resections			
Author, Year	Number of Patients	Number of BSR	%
Todd et al,[23] 1980	67	10	14.8
Wilkins et al,[24] 1984	111	2	1.8
McCaugham et al,[25] 1985	124	52	41.9
Warren et al,[26] 1989	51	9	17.6
Francioni et al,[27] 1990	69	14	21
Schreurs et al,[28] 1992	93	30	32.6
Harpole et al,[29] 1992	126	9	7.14
Marty-Anè et al,[30] 1995	79	10	12.7
Chughtai et al,[31] 1997	84	6	7.14
Ducrocq et al,[32] 1998	139	20	14.4
Carretta et al,[33] 2000	44	3	6.8
Fink et al,[1] 2001	142	2	1.4
Kurul et al,[34] 2002	83	8	9.6
Filosso et al,[35] 2002	126	4	3.2
Mezzetti et al,[36] 2003	98	2	2.0
Cardillo et al,[4] 2004	163	8	4.9
Garcia Yuste[a] et al,[37] 2007	661	66	11.6
Rea et al,[38] 2007	252	32	12.7
Machuca et al,[39] 2010	126	9	7.14
Bagheri et al,[40] 2011	40	5	10.4

Abbreviation: BSR, bronchial sleeve resection.
[a] Retrospective multicenter study.

this operation; however, we can postulate that it can offer survival benefits similar to standard lobectomy. Furthermore, it protects from the detrimental effects of pneumonectomy, which in these young and fit patients should be always avoided. The functional advantages of this approach are evident, as is quality of life. Surgical details are identical to those used in the lung cancer population. Long-term follow-up should rely on the same variables.

In conclusion, bronchoplastic procedures, particularly sleeve resections, are safe in patients with carcinoid tumors and should be the reference for treatment when anatomically and oncologically indicated, independently from pulmonary function.

REFERENCES

1. Fink G, Krelbaum T, Yellin A, et al. Pulmonary carcinoid: presentation, diagnosis and outcome in 142 cases in Israel and review of 640 cases from the literature. Chest 2001;119:1647–51.
2. Detterbeck FC. Management of carcinoid tumors. Ann Thorac Surg 2010;89:998–1005.
3. Hage R, de la Riviere AB, Seldernijk CA, et al. Update on pulmonary carcinoid tumors: a review article. Ann Surg Oncol 2003;10:697–704.
4. Cardillo G, Sera F, Stat D, et al. Bronchial carcinoid tumors: nodal status and long term survival after resection. Ann Thorac Surg 2004;77:1781–5.
5. Travis WD, Rush W, Flieder DB, et al. Survival analysis of 200 pulmonary neuroendocrine tumors with clarification of criteria for atypical carcinoid and its separation from typical carcinoid. Am J Surg Pathol 1998;22:934–44.
6. Cavaliere S, Foccoli P, Toninelli C. Curative bronchoscopic laser therapy for surgically resectable tracheobronchial tumors. J Bronchol 2002;9:90–5.
7. Sutedja TG, Schreurs AJ, Vandershueren RG, et al. Bronchoscopic therapy in patients with intraluminal typical bronchial carcinoid. Chest 1995;107:556–8.
8. Luckraz H, Amer K, Thomas L, et al. Long term outcome of bronchoscopically resected endobronchial typical carcinoid tumors. J Thorac Cardiovasc Surg 2006;132:113–5.
9. Bertoletti L, Ellench R, Kaczmarek D, et al. Bronchoscopic cryotherapy treatment of isolated endoluminal typical carcinoid tumor. Chest 2006;130:1405–11.
10. El Jamal M, Nicholson AG, Goldstraw P. The feasibility of conservative resection for carcinoid tumors: is pneumonectomy ever necessary for uncomplicated cases? Eur J Cardiothorac Surg 2000;18:301–6.
11. Rendina EA, Venuta F, Ciriaco P, et al. Bronchovascular sleeve resection. Technique, preoperative management, prevention and treatment of complications. J Thorac Cardiovasc Surg 1993;106:73–9.
12. Rendina EA, Venuta F, De Giacomo T, et al. Parenchymal sparing operations for bronchogenic carcinoma. Surg Clin North Am 2002;82:589–609.
13. Venuta F, Ciccone AM, Anile M, et al. Reconstruction of the pulmonary artery for lung cancer: long term results. J Thorac Cardiovasc Surg 2009;138:1185–91.
14. Tsubota N. Bronchoplasty at the level of the segmental bronchus. Semin Thorac Cardiovasc Surg 2006;18:96–103.
15. Fu X, Zhang N, Sun W, et al. Multisegmental lobe bronchoplasty for the treatment of non small cell lung cancer. J Huazhong Univ Sci Technolog Med Sci 2007;27:454–6.
16. Okada M, Nishio W, Sakamoto T, et al. Sleeve segmentectomy for non small cell lung carcinoma. J Thorac Cardiovasc Surg 2004;128:420–4.
17. Prince-Thomas C. Conservative resection of the bronchial tree. J R Coll Surg Edinb 1956;1:169–75.
18. Nowak K, Karenovics W, Nicholson AG, et al. Pure bronchoplastic resections of the bronchus without pulmonary resection for endobronchial carcinoid tumors. Interact Cardiovasc Thorac Surg 2013;17:291–4.
19. Lucchi M, Melfi F, Ribechini A, et al. Sleeve and wedge parenchyma sparing bronchial resections in low grade neoplasms of the bronchial airway. J Thorac Cardiovasc Surg 2007;134:373–7.
20. Venuta F, Rendina EA, De Giacomo T, et al. Nd:YAG laser resection of lung cancer invading the airway as a bridge to surgery and palliative treatment. Ann Thorac Surg 2002;74:995–8.
21. Rendina EA, Venuta F, Ricci P, et al. Protection and revascularization of bronchial anastomosis by the intercostal pedicle flap. J Thorac Cardiovasc Surg 1994;107:1251–4.
22. Venuta F, Anile M, Rendina EA. Advantages of the segmental nondivided intercostal pedicle flap. J Thorac Cardiovasc Surg 2010;140:485.
23. Todd TT, Cooper JD, Weissberg D, et al. Bronchial carcinoid tumors. Twenty years' experience. J Thorac Cardiovasc Surg 1980;79:532–6.
24. Wilkins EW Jr, Grillo HC, Moncure AS, et al. Changing times in surgical management of bronchopulmonary carcinoid tumor. Ann Thorac Surg 1984;38:339–44.
25. McCaugham BC, Martini N, Bains MS. Bronchial carcinoids. Review of 124 cses. J Thorac Cardiovasc Surg 1985;89:8–17.
26. Warren WH, Faber LP, Gould VE. Neuroendocrine neoplasms of the lung. A clinicopathologic update. J Thorac Cardiovasc Surg 1989;98:321–32.
27. Francioni F, Rendina EA, Venuta F, et al. Low grade neuroendocrine tumors of the lung (bronchial carcinoids): 25 year experience. Eur J Cardiothorac Surg 1990;4:472–6.
28. Schreurs AJ, Westermann CJ, van den Bosh JM, et al. A twenty-five-year follow up of ninety-three resected typical carcinoid tumors of the lung. J Thorac Cardiovasc Surg 1992;104:1470–5.
29. Harpole DH, Feldman JM, Buchnan S, et al. Bronchial carcinoid tumors: a retrospective analysis of 126 patients. Ann Thorac Surg 1992;54:50–5.

30. Marty-Anè CH, Costes V, Pujol JL, et al. Carcinoid tumors of the lung: do atypical features require aggressive management? Ann Thorac Surg 1995; 59:78–83.

31. Chughtai TS, Morin JE, Sheiner NM, et al. Bronchial carcinoid: twenty years' experience defines a selective surgical approach. Surgery 1997;122:801–8.

32. Ducrocq X, Thomas P, Massard G, et al. Operative risk and prognostic factors of typical bronchial carcinoid tumors. Ann Thorac Surg 1998;65:1410–4.

33. Carretta A, Ceresoli GL, Arrigoni G, et al. Diagnostic and therapeutic management of neuroendocrine lung tumors. A clinical study of 44 cases. Lung Cancer 2000;29:217–25.

34. Kurul IC, Topcu S, Tastepe I, et al. Surgery in bronchial carcinoids: experience with 83 patients. Eur J Cardiothorac Surg 2002;21:883–7.

35. Filosso PL, Rena O, Donati G, et al. Bronchial carcinoid tumors: surgical management and long term outcome. J Thorac Cardiovasc Surg 2002;123: 303–9.

36. Mezzetti M, Raveglia F, Panigalli T, et al. Assessment of outcomes in typical and atypical carcinoids according to the latest WHO classification. Ann Thorac Surg 2003;76:1838–42.

37. Garcia-Yuste M, Matilla JM, Cueto A, et al. Typical and atypical carcinoid tumors: analysis of the experience of the Spanish multi-centric study of neuroendocrine tumours of the lung. Eur J Cardiothorac Surg 2007;31:192–7.

38. Rea F, Rixxardi G, Zuin A, et al. Outcome and surgical strategy in bronchial carcinoid tumors: single institution experience with 252 patients. Eur J Cardiothorac Surg 2007;31:186–91.

39. Machuca TN, Cardoso PF, Camargo SM, et al. Surgical treatment of bronchial carcinoid tumors: a single center experience. Lung Cancer 2010;70:158–62.

40. Bagheri R, Mashhadi MT, Hagi SZ, et al. Tracheobronchopulmonary carcinoid tumors: analysis of 40 patients. Ann Thorac Cardiovasc Surg 2011; 17:7–12.

41. Terzi A, Lonardoni A, Falezza G, et al. Sleeve lobectomy for non small cell lung cancer and carcinoids: in 160 cases. Eur J Cardiothorac Surg 2002;21:888–93.

42. Lemaitri J, Mansour Z, Kochetkowa EA, et al. Bronchoplastic lobectomy: do early results depend on the underlying pathology? A comparison between typical carcinoids and primary lung cancer. Eur J Cardiothorac Surg 2006;30:168–71.

Large-Cell Neuroendocrine Carcinoma of the Lung
Surgical Management

Hiroyuki Sakurai, MD*, Hisao Asamura, MD

KEYWORDS

- Non–small-cell lung cancer • Large-cell neuroendocrine carcinoma • Prognosis

KEY POINTS

- Large-cell neuroendocrine carcinoma (LCNEC) of the lung is an uncommon aggressive neoplasm with a poor prognosis compared with non–small-cell lung carcinoma (NSCLC).
- Because of its rarity, the treatment recommendations for LCNEC are not based on clinical trials, but are extrapolated from the approach to patients with NSCLC and small-cell lung carcinoma and the established literature for LCNEC, which is primarily retrospective in nature.
- Further studies should clarify the histology-specific characteristic and optimal therapeutic approach to establish the entity of LCNEC.

INTRODUCTION

Large-cell neuroendocrine carcinoma (LCNEC) of the lung is a relatively uncommon and aggressive subset of non–small-cell carcinomas (NSCLC), within the spectrum of pulmonary neuroendocrine tumors, which include typical and atypical carcinoid, and small-cell lung cancer (SCLC).[1–3] LCNECs were first reported by Travis and colleagues[4] in 1991 as a separate category of pulmonary neuroendocrine tumors, distinct from typical and atypical carcinoids and SCLC. They described LCNECs as tumors composed of large cells characterized by a light microscopic neuroendocrine appearance with a low nuclear-to-cytoplasmic ratio, frequent nucleoli, a high mitotic rate (greater than 10 mitoses per 10 high-power fields), and abundant necrosis, in addition to neuroendocrine differentiation detected by electron microscopy or immunohistochemistry.[4] In the 1999 World Health Organization (WHO) classification,[5] these pathologic features were adopted as criteria for the LCNEC diagnosis.

LCNEC of the lung is considered to be very aggressive, and clinical outcome is poorer than expected for stage-matched NSCLC, similar to the dismal outcome of SCLC, with 5-year survival rates ranging between 15% and 60%.[3,6–8] Therefore, considerable debate has emerged about whether these tumors should be treated or considered together with SCLC. However, the reported prognoses are heterogeneous and the optimum treatment has not yet been identified. Here we review the pertinent literature on resected LCNEC of the lung, and examine its clinicopathological features and prognosis.

CLINICAL CHARACTERISTICS

Although not well defined, the incidence of LCNEC in primary lung cancers is likely very low. Since Jiang and colleagues[9] reported that 22 (2.8%) of 766 resected primary lung cancers were classified as LCNEC, several investigators reported similar rates. Based on the available literature, the incidence of LCNEC among resected lung cancers appears to be between 2.1% and 3.5%.[10–12]

Division of Thoracic Surgery, National Cancer Center Hospital, 5-1-1 Tsukiji, Chuo-ku, Tokyo 104-0045, Japan
* Corresponding author.
E-mail address: hsakurai@ncc.go.jp

thoracic.theclinics.com

Men most commonly comprise 80% to 90% of patients with LCNEC[7,11,13]: Sarkaria and colleagues[14] reported 54% men in the Memorial LCNEC series. More than 85% of patients have a history of cigarette smoking[7,11,15]; therefore, smoking appears to be the primary cause in LCNEC development. The median age of patients ranged between 62 and 68 years.[7,12,14,16,17]

Regarding the tumor location, LCNECs mostly present as peripheral tumors,[3,18] as opposed to the central carcinoids and SCLC site, and therefore clinical symptoms are less commonly detected. Garcia-Yuste and colleagues[19] reported that two-thirds of LCNECs presented in the pulmonary parenchyma periphery. A computed tomography appearance generally shows a well-defined and lobulated nodule/mass that resembles that of other expansively growing tumors, such as peripheral SCLC, poorly differentiated adenocarcinomas, and squamous cell carcinomas (**Fig. 1**).[20–23] Regarding 2-[^{18}F]-fluoro-2-deoxy-D-glucose positron-emission tomography findings, Kaira and colleagues[24] reported that the standardized uptake value peek was significantly higher in LCNEC as well as SCLC, than in carcinoid, with a mean value of 13.7.[24]

Paraneoplastic and ectopic hormone production syndromes have been very infrequently observed and occasionally reported by Travis and colleagues,[25] Paci and colleagues,[18] Asamura and colleagues,[7] Takei and colleagues,[11] and Zacharias and colleagues.[26] Among serum tumor markers measured before surgery, the carcinoembryonic antigen and progastrin-releasing peptide, which is a good marker of high-grade neuroendocrine

tumors such as SCLS, seem to be relatively elevated in patients with LCNEC (**Table 1**).[7,10,11]

Additionally, Sarkaria and colleagues[14] observed how LCNEC has a comparatively high incidence (21%) of prior nonlung cancers.

It is difficult to diagnose LCNECs from preoperative biopsies, although cytologic characteristics have been carefully studied.[27–29] LCNECs have been usually diagnosed in surgical specimens, postoperatively.

PATHOLOGY

Neuroendocrine tumors of the lung are a distinct subset of tumors that share definite morphologic, ultrastructural, immunohistochemical, and molecular characteristics.[30] Additionally, they encompass a spectrum of low-grade typical carcinoid, intermediate-grade atypical carcinoid, and high-grade LCNEC and SCLC.[25] Mitotic activity is the most important criterion to establish tumor type.

Immunohistochemical markers offer the most reliable means to detect neuroendocrine differentiation. Neuroendocrine tumors are identified by the presence of one or more of the following neuroendocrine markers: chromogranin A, synaptophysin, and neural cell adhesion molecule (NCAM).[5] Rossi and colleagues[31] first described the percentage of chromogranin A (65%), synaptophysin (53%), and NCAM (93%) in LCNEC. Evidence of neuroendocrine differentiation also can be ultrastructurally achieved through electron microscopy. Rusch and colleagues[32] identified the patterns of expression of several molecular markers in pulmonary neuroendocrine tumors. The investigators showed that Ki-67, p53, and Rb expression could be useful to distinguish LCNEC and SCLC from typical and atypical carcinoids.[32] Moreover, LCNEC and SCLC show a higher Ki-67 proliferation rate, abnormal p53, and the lack of Rb staining in comparison with typical and atypical carcinoids.[32]

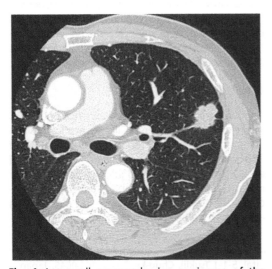

Fig. 1. Large-cell neuroendocrine carcinoma of the lung on high-resolution computed tomography. The tumor shows a well-defined lobulated nodule at the periphery in the left upper lobe of the lung.

Table 1			
Percentage of preoperative elevation of serum tumor markers (CEA, NSE, and proGRP) for large cell neuroendocrine carcinoma			
Author (Year)	**CEA (%)**	**NSE (%)**	**proGRP (%)**
Iyoda et al,[10] 2001	34.0	34.1	—
Takei et al,[11] 2002	49.0	19.0	11.0
Asamura et al,[7] 2006	48.5	12.4	25.8

Abbreviations: CEA, carcinoembryonic antigen; NSE, neuron-specific enolase; proGRP, progastrin-releasing peptide.
Data from Refs.[7,10,11]

Additional molecular analysis might elucidate a role of targeted therapies for LCNEC.[30]

Histologic LCNEC characteristics include large cell type (at least 3 times larger than SCLC), low nuclear-to-cytoplasmic ratio, high mitotic rate and necrosis, in addition to neuroendocrine morphology. The criteria for a correct LCNEC diagnosis, based on the recent WHO classification[5] are (1) neuroendocrine morphology (organoid nesting, palisading, rosettes, trabeculae), (2) high mitotic rate (11 or more per 2 mm^2 in 10 high-power fields), (3) necrosis, (4) cytologic features of a NSCLC, and (5) positive immunohistochemical staining for 1 or more neuroendocrine markers and/or neuroendocrine granules by electron microscopy. A preoperative diagnosis of LCNEC, based on small biopsies or cytology, is very difficult because of the problems identifying the neuroendocrine morphology and demonstrating neuroendocrine differentiation by immunohistochemistry in a small tissue sample.[8]

On the other hand, LCNEC is considered to be a variant of large-cell carcinoma according to the Third WHO classification.[5] Large-cell carcinomas (LCCs) are, in fact, divided into the following 4 types according to neuroendocrine features: (1) LCNEC, (2) large-cell carcinoma with neuroendocrine differentiation (LCCND), large-cell carcinoma with a neuroendocrine morphology (LCCNM), and classic large-cell carcinoma (CLCC).[5] The diagnostic criteria for these tumors are shown in **Table 2**. As reported by Iyoda and colleagues[10] on 199 cases of LCC, 50 (42%) were classified as LCNEC, 9 (7.6%) as LCCND, 13 (10.9%) as LCCNM, and 47 (39.5%) as CLCC. Additionally, the overall survival for patients with LCC with neuroendocrine features, such as LCNEC, LCCND, and LCCNM, was significantly shorter than that for patients with CLCC.[10] The clinical behavior of LCCND and LCCNM is likely to be similar to that of LCNEC.[28,33]

When LCNECs are accompanied by other histologies (squamous cell, spindle cell carcinoma) they are called combined LCNEC. Approximately 10% to 20% of surgically resected LCNECs are combined.[1,7,10] The commonest associated histologic subtype is adenocarcinoma.[10] If SCLC is coexistent with LCNEC, the tumor is diagnosed as a combined SCLC.[5]

SURVIVAL

The 5-year overall survival rate in patients with resected LCNEC has been reported to range between 13% and 57% for all stages,[34] and between 18% and 88% for patients with stage 1 (**Table 3**).[6,7,9–12,14,16,18,19,25,26,35–37] This difference is probably due to the small number of patients with LCNEC included in each report or an imprecise pathologic diagnosis of LCNEC. Asamura and colleagues[7] reported outcomes of surgically resected pulmonary neuroendocrine tumors including 141 LCNECs, the histologic diagnosis of which was reviewed by a pathology panel consisting of 6 expert pathologists. According to this report, the survival curves of patients with LCNEC and SCLC were superimposed and far worse than those of the patients with bronchial carcinoid, with 5-year survival rates of 40% and 36% for LCNEC and SCLC, compared with 96% and 78% for typical and atypical carcinoids. In many series, patients with resected LCNEC have worse survival compared with those with LCC or other NSCLCs,[12,38,39] even in stage 1.[12,37] LCNEC survival rates are almost similar to SCLC rates.[7,25,40–42] These 2 histologies share a similar clinicopathologic background, including smoking history and predominant male sex. Asamura and colleagues[7] found that an LCNEC histology was an independent predictor of a poor prognosis, as supported by other researchers.[12,17,37]

Combined LCNECs appear to behave as LCNEC rather than LCC.[8,14] Battafarano and

Table 2
Typing of large-cell carcinoma according to neuroendocrine features

Diagnosis	Neuroendocrine Morphology	Neuroendocrine Features on Immunohistochemistry or Electron Microscopy
LCNEC	Yes	Yes
LCCNM	Yes	No
LCCND	No	Yes
CLCC	No	No

Abbreviations: CLCC, classic large cell carcinoma; LCCND, large cell carcinoma with neuroendocrine differentiation; LCCNM, large cell carcinoma with neuroendocrine morphology; LCNEC, large cell neuroendocrine carcinoma.

Adapted from Lim E, Goldstraw P, Nicholson AG, et al. Proceedings of the IASLC international workshop on advances in pulmonary neuroendocrine tumors 2007. J Thorac Oncol 2008;3:1195; with permission.

Table 3
Postoperative 5-year survival rates for patients with large cell neuroendocrine carcinoma of the lung

Author (Year)	No. of Patients	5-Year Survival Rate (All) (%)	5-Year Survival Rate (Each Stage)
Dresler et al,[35] 1997	40	13.0	Stage 1 (n = 25), 18%
Travis et al,[25] 1998	37	27.0	—
Jiang et al,[9] 1998	17	44.8	—
Garcia-Yuste et al,[19] 2000	22	20.8	Stage 1, 33%
Iyoda et al,[10] 2001	50	35.3	—
Takei et al,[11] 2002	87	57.0	Stage 1 (n = 41)/2 (n = 13)/3 (n = 30), 67%/75%/45%
Skuladottir et al,[6] 2002	50	15.0	—
Zacharias et al,[26] 2003	21	47.0	Stage 1 (n = 9)/2–3 (n = 9), 88%/28%
Paci et al,[18] 2004	48	21.2	Stage 1 (n = 29)/2 (n = 11)/3 (n = 8), 27.0%/18.1%/0%
Doddoli et al,[36] 2004	20	36.0	Stage 1–2 (n = 8)/3–4 (n = 12), 54%/25%
Battafarano et al,[12] 2005	45	30.3	Stage 1 (n = 30), 33.3%
Iyoda et al,[37] 2006	11	—	Stage 1A (n = 11), 54.5%
Asamura et al,[7] 2006	141	40.3	Stage 1 (n = 63), 60%
Veronesi et al,[16] 2006	144	43.0	Stage 1 (n = 73)/2 (n = 29)/3 (n = 40), 52%/59%/20%
Sarkaria et al,[14] 2011	100	—	Stage 1A (n = 26)/1B (n = 18), 72%/26%

colleagues[12] showed that they behave poorly, with a 5-year overall survival rate of 30%. Therefore, the presence of neuroendocrine features in any portion of the tumor appears to be associated with poor prognosis. Additionally, Iyoda and colleagues[10] investigated the difference in the clinico-biological behavior of 4 LCC types (LCNEC, LCCND, LCCNM, and CLCC), based on their neuroendocrine features. The clinical behaviors of LCCNM and LCCND were similar to LCNEC, and these 3 types of LCC presented a worse outcome compared with CLCC.[10] Because LCC with any degree of neuroendocrine features shows a very aggressive biology, the pathology of LCC should be examined carefully for evidence of occult neuroendocrine features.

On a multivariate analysis, male gender, high age, advanced stage, and pneumonectomy have been reported to be negative prognostic factors.[1,14,16] According Faggiano and colleagues,[43] high mitotic count (>37 per 10 high-power fields) and less than 2 immunohistochemically positive neuroendocrine markers were independent negative pathologic variables. Nevertheless, Takei and colleagues[11] described that there was no correlation between the pattern of staining of neuroendocrine markers and survival.

Tumor recurrences usually develop early, even after a complete tumor resection. Iyoda and colleagues[17] reported that 64% of them occur within

1 year after surgery and 91% within 3 years; Takei and colleagues[11] observed 82% and 91% recurrences after 1 and 2 years, respectively. Most patients (56%–60%) present with distant metastases.[7,11,17]

TREATMENT

Treatment options for patients with LCNEC are based on the extrapolation from the approach to patients with NSCLC. Therefore, in stage 1 or 2 LCNEC, surgical resection is indicated whenever feasible. Because the prognosis is worse, adjuvant chemotherapy may improve survival, as suggested by several studies.[1,14,17] However, as a result of the small number of patients in each study and the relative infrequency of LCNEC, no standard adjuvant therapy regimen has been developed.[1,21] In a retrospective analysis of 83 patients, Rossi and colleagues[31] found significantly improved outcomes in those who received adjuvant SCLC-based therapy (cisplatin/etoposide) versus those who received platinum regimens in combination with other agents. In a small prospective, nonrandomized, single-arm trial, Iyoda and colleagues[44] reported 88.9% 5-year survival rate in patients receiving adjuvant cisplatin-etoposide versus 47.4% in those who did not. Disease-free survival and recurrence rates were also significantly better in patients who received chemotherapy. This is the only prospective trial on adjuvant therapy, and the investigators concluded demonstrating the efficacy of adjuvant chemotherapy in such rare tumors.[44]

A recent meta-analysis showed that a cisplatin/irinotecan regimen may be an alternative to a cisplatin/etoposide regimen as first-line treatment in SCLC.[45,46] Thus, a prospective, randomized, multi-institutional phase III trial is currently being conducted by the Japan Clinical Oncology Group to compare cisplatin/etoposide to cisplatin/irinotecan in the setting of adjuvant chemotherapy for resected LCNEC. The role of neoadjuvant therapy has not yet been studied.[14]

Finally, there has also been a report on octreotide efficacy as adjuvant treatment in resected LCNEC.[47] Octreotide is a long-acting synthetic somatostatin analog that inhibits the secretion of a broad range of hormones, such as growth hormone, insulin, glucagon, and gastrin. Its antitumoral effect has been demonstrated in vitro[48] but the utility of octreotide in patients with LCNEC remains controversial.

SUMMARY

LCNEC of the lung is an uncommon aggressive neoplasm with a poor prognosis compared with NSCLC. Because of its rarity, the treatment recommendations are not based on clinical trials, but are extrapolated from the approach to patients with NSCLC and SCLC and the established literature for LCNEC, which is primarily retrospective in nature. Further studies should clarify the histology-specific characteristic and optimal therapeutic approach to establish the entity of LCNEC.

REFERENCES

1. Lim E, Goldstraw P, Nicholson AG, et al. Proceedings of the IASLC international workshop on advances in pulmonary neuroendocrine tumors 2007. J Thorac Oncol 2008;3:1194–201.
2. Shields TW. Pathology of carcinoma of the lung. In: Shields TW, LoCicero J, Reed CE, et al, editors. General thoracic surgery. 7th edition. Philadelphia: Lippincott Williams and Wilkins; 2009. p. 1311–40.
3. Glisson BS, Moran CA. Large-cell neuroendocrine carcinoma: controversies in diagnosis and treatment. J Natl Compr Canc Netw 2011;9:1122–9.
4. Travis WD, Linnoila RI, Tsokos MG, et al. Neuroendocrine tumors of the lung with proposed criteria for large-cell neuroendocrine carcinoma. An ultrastructural, immunohistochemical, and flow cytometric study of 35 cases. Am J Surg Pathol 1991;15:529–53.
5. Travis WD, Colby TV, Corrin B, et al. Histological typing of lung and pleural tumours, World Health Organization International Histological Classification of Tumors. Berlin: Springer; 1999.
6. Skuladottir H, Hirsch FR, Hansen HH, et al. Pulmonary neuroendocrine tumors: incidence and prognosis of histological subtypes. A population-based study in Denmark. Lung Cancer 2002;37:127–35.
7. Asamura H, Kameya T, Matsuno Y, et al. Neuroendocrine neoplasms of the lung: a prognostic spectrum. J Clin Oncol 2006;24:70–6.
8. Fernandez FG, Battafarano RJ. Large-cell neuroendocrine carcinoma of the lung: an aggressive neuroendocrine lung cancer. Semin Thorac Cardiovasc Surg 2006;18:206–10.
9. Jiang SX, Kameya T, Shoji M, et al. Large cell neuroendocrine carcinoma of the lung. A histologic and immunohistochemical study of 22 cases. Am J Surg Pathol 1998;22:526–37.
10. Iyoda A, Hiroshima K, Toyozaki T, et al. Clinical characterization of pulmonary large cell neuroendocrine carcinoma and large cell carcinoma with neuroendocrine morphology. Cancer 2001;91:1992–2000.
11. Takei H, Asamura H, Maeshima A, et al. Large cell neuroendocrine carcinoma of the lung: a clinicopathologic study of eighty-seven cases. J Thorac Cardiovasc Surg 2002;124:285–92.
12. Battafarano RJ, Fernandez FG, Ritter J, et al. Large call neuroendocrine carcinoma: an aggressive form of non-small cell lung cancer. J Thorac Cardiovasc Surg 2005;130:166–72.
13. Grand B, Cazes A, Mordant P, et al. High grade neuroendocrine lung tumors: pathological characteristics, surgical management and prognostic implications. Lung Cancer 2013;81:404–9.
14. Sarkaria IS, Iyoda A, Roh MS, et al. Neoadjuvant and adjuvant chemotherapy in resected pulmonary large cell neuroendocrine carcinomas: a single institution experience. Ann Thorac Surg 2011;92:1180–7.
15. Hage R, Seldenrijk K, de Bruin P, et al. Pulmonary large-cell neuroendocrine carcinoma (LCNEC). Eur J Cardiothorac Surg 2003;23:457–60.
16. Veronesi G, Morandi U, Alloisio M, et al. Large cell neuroendocrine carcinoma of the lung: a retrospective analysis of 144 surgical cases. Lung Cancer 2006;53:111–5.
17. Iyoda A, Hiroshima K, Moriya Y, et al. Postoperative recurrence and the role of adjuvant chemotherapy in patients with pulmonary large-cell neuroendocrine carcinoma. J Thorac Cardiovasc Surg 2009;138:446–53.
18. Paci M, Cavazza A, Annessi V, et al. Large cell neuroendocrine carcinoma of the lung: a 10-year clinicopathologic retrospective study. Ann Thorac Surg 2004;77:1163–7.
19. Garcia-Yuste M, Matilla JM, Alvarez-Gago T, et al. Prognostic factors in neuroendocrine lung tumors: a Spanish multicenter study. Ann Thorac Surg 2000;70:258–63.

20. Shin AR, Shin BK, Choi JA, et al. Large cell neuroendocrine carcinoma of the lung: radiologic and pathologic findings. J Comput Assist Tomogr 2000;24: 567–73.

21. Jung KJ, Lee KS, Han J, et al. Large cell neuroendocrine carcinoma of the lung: clinical, CT, and pathologic findings in 11 patients. J Thorac Imaging 2001; 16:156–62.

22. Oshiro Y, Kusumoto M, Matsuno Y, et al. CT findings of surgically resected large cell neuroendocrine carcinoma of the lung in 38 patients. AJR Am J Roentgenol 2004;182:87–91.

23. Akata S, Okada S, Maeda J, et al. Computed tomographic findings of large cell neuroendocrine carcinoma of the lung. Clin Imaging 2007;31:379–84.

24. Kaira K, Murakami H, Endo M, et al. Biological correlation of 18F-FDG uptake on PET in pulmonary neuroendocrine tumors. Anticancer Res 2013;33: 4219–28.

25. Travis WD, Rush W, Flieder DB, et al. Survival analysis of 200 pulmonary neuroendocrine tumors with clarification of criteria for atypical carcinoid and its separation from typical carcinoid. Am J Surg Pathol 1998;22:934–44.

26. Zacharias J, Nicholson AG, Ladas GP, et al. Large cell neuroendocrine carcinoma and large cell carcinomas with neuroendocrine morphology of the lung: prognosis after complete resection and systemic nodal dissection. Ann Thorac Surg 2003;75:348–52.

27. Hiroshima K, Abe S, Ebihara Y, et al. Cytological characteristics of pulmonary large cell neuroendocrine carcinoma. Lung Cancer 2005;48:331–7.

28. Iyoda A, Hiroshima K, Nakatani Y, et al. Pulmonary large cell neuroendocrine carcinoma: its place in the spectrum of pulmonary carcinoma. Ann Thorac Surg 2007;84:702–7.

29. Maleki Z. Diagnostic issues with cytopathologic interpretation of lung neoplasms displaying high-grade basaloid or neuroendocrine morphology. Diagn Cytopathol 2011;39:159–67.

30. Iyoda A, Travis W, Sarkaria IS, et al. Expression profiling and identification of potential molecular targets for therapy in pulmonary large-cell neuroendocrine carcinoma. Exp Ther Med 2011;2:1041–5.

31. Rossi G, Cavazza A, Marchioni A, et al. Role of chemotherapy and the receptor tyrosine kinases KIT, PDGFRα, PDGFRβ, and Met in large-cell neuroendocrine carcinoma of the lung. J Clin Oncol 2005; 23:8774–85.

32. Rusch VW, Klimstra DS, Venkatraman ES. Molecular markers help characterize neuroendocrine lung tumors. Ann Thorac Surg 1996;62:798–810.

33. Peng WX, Sano T, Oyama T, et al. Large cell neuroendocrine carcinoma of the lung: a comparison with large cell carcinoma with neuroendocrine morphology and small cell carcinoma. Lung Cancer 2005;47:225–33.

34. International Union Against Cancer. Lung and pleural tumours. In: Sobin LH, Gospodarowicz M, editors. TNM classification of malignant tumours. 7th edition. New York: Wiley-Blackwell; 2009. p. 138–46.

35. Dresler CM, Ritter JH, Patterson GA, et al. Clinical-pathologic analysis of 40 patients with large cell neuroendocrine carcinoma of the lung. Ann Thorac Surg 1997;63:180–5.

36. Doddoli C, Barlesi F, Chetaille B, et al. Large cell neuroendocrine carcinoma of the lung: an aggressive disease potentially treatable with surgery. Ann Thorac Surg 2004;77:1168–72.

37. Iyoda A, Hiroshima K, Moriya Y, et al. Prognostic impact of large cell neuroendocrine histology in patents with pathologic Ia pulmonary non-small cell carcinoma. J Thorac Cardiovasc Surg 2006; 132:312–5.

38. Iyoda A, Hiroshima K, Moriya Y, et al. Pulmonary large cell neuroendocrine carcinoma demonstrates high proliferative activity. Ann Thorac Surg 2004; 77:1891–5.

39. Ab'Saber AM, Neto LM, Bianchi CP, et al. Neuroendocrine and biologic features of primary tumors and tissue in pulmonary large cell carcinomas. Ann Thorac Surg 2004;77:1883–90.

40. Isaka M, Nakagawa K, Ohde Y, et al. A clinicopathological study of peripheral, small-sized high-grade neuroendocrine tumours of the lung: differences between small-cell lung carcinoma and large-cell neuroendocrine carcinoma. Eur J Cardiothorac Surg 2012;41:841–6.

41. Kinoshita T, Yoshida J, Ishii G, et al. The differences of biological behavior based on the clinicopathological data between resectable large-cell neuroendocrine and small-cell lung carcinoma. Clin Lung Cancer 2013;14:535–40.

42. Cooper WA, Thourani VH, Gal AA, et al. The surgical spectrum of pulmonary neuroendocrine neoplasms. Chest 2001;119:14–8.

43. Faggiano A, Sabourin JC, Ducreux M, et al. Pulmonary and extrapulmonary poorly differentiated large cell neuroendocrine carcinomas. Diagnostic and prognostic features. Cancer 2007;110:265–74.

44. Iyoda A, Hiroshima K, Moriya Y, et al. Prospective study of adjuvant chemotherapy for pulmonary large cell neuroendocrine carcinoma. Ann Thorac Surg 2006;82:1802–7.

45. Jiang J, Liang X, Zhou X, et al. A meta-analysis of randomized controlled trials comparing irinotecan/platinum with etoposide/platinum in patients with previously untreated extensive-stage small cell lung cancer. J Thorac Oncol 2010;5:867–73.

46. Niho S, Kenmotsu H, Sekine I, et al. Combination chemotherapy with irinotecan and cisplatin for large-cell neuroendocrine carcinoma of the lung. A multicenter phase II study. J Thorac Oncol 2013;8: 980–4.

47. Filosso PL, Ruffini E, Oliaro A, et al. Large-cell neuro-endocrine carcinoma of the lung: a clinicopathologic study of eighteen cases and the efficacy of adjuvant treatment with octreotide. J Thorac Cardiovasc Surg 2005;129:819–24.

48. Taylor JE, Bogden AE, Moreau JP, et al. In vitro and in vivo inhabitation of human small cell lung carcinoma (NCI-H69) growth by a somatostatin analogue. Biochem Biophys Res Commun 1998; 153:81–6.

Neuroendocrine Tumors of the Lung
The Role of Surgery in Small Cell Lung Cancer

Georgios Stamatis, MD

KEYWORDS

- Staging • Indications • Surgery • Results • Small cell lung cancer

KEY POINTS

- The role of surgical treatment in the management of patients with small cell lung cancer (SCLC) remains controversial.
- Although in the past, 2 randomized studies have failed to show any benefit on survival by adding surgery to chemotherapy (CTx), different retrospective and prospective reports, including the recently published studies using the database of the Cancer Institute Surveillance Epidemiology and End Results, showed that surgery offers a reasonable overall survival in a subset of patients with stage I and II SCLC.
- Two important recommendations have been introduced concerning SCLC histology as a high-grade aggressive neuroendocrine tumor and the use of TNM classification in SCLC staging and in clinical trials.
- Patients' selection is fundamental, and it should include extensive radiologic staging and mediastinal lymph-node biopsy.
- The use of a positron emission tomography scan is likely to improve the accuracy of staging.
- Through primary surgery or after induction CTx, a complete tumor resection associated with systematic hilar/mediastinal lymphadenectomy should be achieved.
- Adjuvant CTx is also recommended in patients with stage I disease; prophylactic cranial irradiation prolongs survival in those patients who achieve a complete or partial response to initial treatment.
- Surgery can be performed with a curative intent in patients with stage I or II disease or significant nodal response after CTx.

INTRODUCTION

Small cell lung cancer (SCLC) represents a distinct pathologic and clinical entity, accounting for approximately 10% to 20% of all primary lung cancers, with incidence rates declining in men but continuing to increase in women in most countries.[1,2] SCLC is the most aggressive among lung cancer subtypes: it has a poor prognosis and is closely associated with smoking history. Regional lymph node involvement or distant metastasis is present in more than 90% of patients at the time of diagnosis.[3] The Veterans Administration Surgical Oncology Group (VASOG) has introduced a simple staging system to be used in their clinical trials, dividing SCLC into 2 disease subgroups termed *limited disease* (LD) and *extensive disease* (ED). LD-SCLC was defined as a disease that can

The author has nothing to disclose.
Department of Thoracic Surgery and Endoscopy, Ruhrlandklinik, West German Lung Center, University of Duisburg-Essen, Tueschenerweg 40, Essen 45239, Germany
E-mail address: georgios.stamatis@ruhrlandklinik.uk-essen.de

Thorac Surg Clin 24 (2014) 313–326
http://dx.doi.org/10.1016/j.thorsurg.2014.05.004
1547-4127/14/$ – see front matter © 2014 Elsevier Inc. All rights reserved.

thoracic.theclinics.com

potentially be encompassed within a tolerable radiation field. Tumor extension is limited to the hemithorax, including regional and ipsilateral supraclavicular nodes. ED-SCLC was classified as a disease outside of these confines.[4]

Two important recommendations have been introduced in the last decade concerning SCLC histology and its TNM classification: (1) In 1999, the World Health Organization's classification of lung and pleural tumors recognized SCLC as a high-grade, biologically aggressive neuroendocrine tumor with a different immunohistochemical and morphologic appearance, different from typical and atypical carcinoid, and large cell neuroendocrine carcinoma.[5] (2) In 2007, the International Association for Study of Lung Cancer (IASLC), using the IASLC database of 8088 SCLC cases, performed a survival analysis for clinically staged patients. Prognostic groups were compared, and the new IASLC TNM proposals were applied to this population and to the Surveillance, Epidemiology, and End Results (SEER) database. This analysis demonstrated the clinical TNM staging utility for this malignancy, so that TNM staging is now recommended for SCLC and stratification by stage I to IIIA should be incorporated in clinical trials or early disease.[6,7]

Surgery was the treatment choice of in the 1960s, but the reported cases showed a generally worse prognosis compared with other lung cancer subtypes.[8,9] The introduction of chemotherapy (CTx) and the results of a randomized study organized by the British Medical Research Council, published by Fox, highlighted the dogma that surgery alone is not the optimal treatment of patients with SCLC.[10] In this study, 144 patients were randomized: 71 to surgery and 73 to radiotherapy. The median survival time in the surgery group was 199 days versus 300 days in the radiotherapy one; the 5-year survival rates were 1.4% and 4.1%, respectively. Although the observation that radiotherapy was superior to surgery, the overall results of both arms seemed to be very poor. However, this study has been criticized for many reasons; the poor survival after surgery might be related to the fact that histologic diagnosis was based on results from rigid bronchoscopy, so that only patients with centrally located tumors were eligible for this study. Moreover, the patients were not staged using the modern technical standards (computed tomography scan, mediastinoscopy, 2-Fluor-2-desoxy-D-glucose (FDG)–positron emission tomography [PET], and so forth), and intraoperative staging was not complete because mediastinal lymph-nodal dissection was generally not performed.[11]

Systemic CTx was then introduced for the treatment of SCLC and resulted in objective response rates of 80%, palliation of symptoms, and prolonged survival.[12] Despite this, long-term survival remained disappointing: According to the initial disease extent, long-term survival rates did not exceed 10% to 15% in LD-SCLC. In 537 of such patients, who received various protocols of intensive CTx or chemoradiotherapy combination with complete clinical response, Elliott and colleagues[13] identified, at autopsy, a residual tumor at the primary site in 64% and in hilar and mediastinal lymph nodes in 53%.

Therefore, strategies to improve outcomes have included CTx concurrently with radiation or have tried intensification of radiotherapy as early as possible.

A major systemic risk for long-term SCLC survivors is the brain metastasis development. A careful meta-analysis of published randomized trials demonstrated a significant effect of prophylactic cranial irradiation (PCI) on survival in patients with LD and complete response.[14]

In 1989, the Toronto Lung Oncology Group published encouraging results with a prospective study of adjuvant surgical resection after CTx for LD-SCLC. They found that adjuvant surgical treatment significantly contributed to improved survival for patients with stage I disease (N0 tumors and tumors of mixed histology). They emphasized the importance of intensive preoperative staging, including mediastinoscopy for possible candidates to adjuvant surgery as definitive local treatment.[15]

To determine the role of surgery in combination with CTx and radiotherapy, with the aim to prolong survival and improve the cure rates, the Lung Cancer Study Group in cooperation with the Eastern Cooperative Oncology Group and the European Organization for Research and Treatment of Cancer started a prospective randomized trial of adjuvant surgical resection. Patients received 5 cycles of CTx with cyclophosphamide, doxorubicin, vincristine, and etoposide; in absence of toxicity or progressive disease, they were restaged and functionally evaluated for possible thoracotomy. Eligible patients were randomized, either to surgical resection followed by thoracic radiation and PCI or to radiotherapy and PCI without surgery. One hundred forty-four patients were randomized: 68 received surgery followed by radiotherapy and 76 radiotherapy alone. Only 54 out of the operated patients had a pathologic complete resection (R0). The median overall survival time was 14 months and 18 months for the randomized patients. There was no significant difference in median or overall survival between the two randomizations.[16] However, different aspects of this study have been criticized. Pathologic staging was available for the group of patients who underwent surgery only; pretreatment or preoperative staging was suboptimal according to the modern standards. Thoracic computed tomography scan was not always performed in the pretreatment setting, and preoperative diagnosis was achieved through bronchoscopy or mediastinoscopy. Consequently, only patients with centrally located lesions or those with extensive mediastinal disease were included.

Resectability criteria were not well defined, so patients with bulky N2 disease could be initially enrolled, whereas only those with supraclavicular nodes or with neoplastic pleural effusions were excluded.[17]

Shields and colleagues[18] first pointed out the importance of the TNM staging system also for SCLC and reported 5-year survival rates of about 59.5% in pathologic stage T1N0M0, 31.3% in T1N1M0, and 27.9% in T2N0M0.[18] In patients with T1 or T2 lesions with negative mediastinal exploration, initial surgical resection followed by an adequate CTx and PCI has resulted in an 80% disease-free survival at 30 months.[19] These observations suggested the existence of a small group of LD-SCLC in which surgery in combination with systemic CTx might be effective.

Recently, different studies using the SEER database analyzed the outcomes of 3566 patients with SCLC stage I and II from 1988 to 2007. The surgical treatment was performed in 895 patients (25.1%); the median survival was 34 months in the surgical group versus 16 months in the nonsurgical group.[20] In a similar report by Yu and colleagues,[21] the 5-year overall survival was 21.1%, but it was 50.3% for those patients who received a resection (45.7% after pneumonectomy and 33.7% after sublobar one). This analysis confirmed the acceptable survival rates in a subset of patients with stage I SCLC.

Until now, the standard systemic treatment of patients with LD-SCLC remains the combination of platinum and etoposide. Several targeted agents have been investigated in LD and ED-SCLC, mostly in unselected populations, with disappointing results.[22] A large randomized study has failed to show any benefit from the addition of thalidomide to traditional CTx.[23] Taking into account the TNM use in SCLC, the encouraging SEER results for patients submitted to surgery, as well as the development of new effective drugs for systemic treatment, a reconsideration of the role of surgery seems to be mandatory.

Consequently, the aim of this report is to investigate the impact of stage on survival in stage I to IIIA SCLC, after surgery alone and as part of multimodality approach, with the review of the previous and current clinical series published in the literature.

RATIONALE FOR SURGERY
Suspicious Pulmonary Lesions

Accurate stage provides prognostic information and aids for the treatment strategy planning in all lung cancer subtypes. Historically, the best results in terms of survival for T1 to T2 tumors can be achieved by surgery alone.[24,25] Maassen and colleagues[26] reported that 25% of patients with SCLC who underwent resection did not have a histologic diagnosis before operation. In peripheral clinical N0 tumors without metastatic disease, up-front surgery can be performed, followed by CTx or CTx-RTx (radiotherapy) and PCI. Although only 5% of patients with SCLC initially present with stage I disease, the increasing use of computed tomography imaging and the trend to remove suspicious lung lesions through minimal invasive thoracoscopic procedures without prior histologic or cytologic examination may increase the number of early stage SCLC in the future.[27]

Improved Local Control

Because of the tendency to early metastasize, systemic CTx has been the cornerstone of treatment also in limited disease; objective response rates varied between 80% and 100%.[28] Long-term survival improvement of up to 20% can be achieved by early inclusion of thoracic irradiation.[29,30] However, even in modern chemoradiation protocols, many patients experience tumor recurrences, either local or distant.[31] A meta-analysis of 3.681 patients treated with CTx, published by the Lung Cancer Subcommittee of the United Kingdom Coordinating Committee for Cancer Research, showed a 2-year survival of 5.9% for patients overall, 8.5% for LD-SCLC, and 2.2% for ED-SCLC.[32] A pattern of relapse analysis in patients with LD showed that local recurrences were the most common cause for failure.[33]

Two thoracic radiotherapy meta-analyses published in 1992 reported data about local control in 2000 patients with SCLC. The inclusion of aggressive radiation techniques after CTx resulted in a significant improvement of local control and a decrease in local recurrence rate of 25%. The median overall survival time was longer than 20 months, and a 5-year survival rate of approximately 20% was also reported. Despite these encouraging results, local relapses were observed in 25% of the patients, with an approximately 50% cumulative risk.[31,34,35]

Recently, 3 different studies analyzed the SEER database to evaluate stage I to III outcomes in patients treated between 1988 and 2004.[20,21] A total of 14.179 patients were studied, including 863 who underwent surgical resection. The median overall survival was 34 months in surgical patients versus 16 month in the nonsurgical group. Surgery was significantly associated with an improved median survival for both localized and regional disease (15–42 vs 12–22 months, respectively). Surgery also improved median survival in N0, N1, and N2 disease.[36]

These findings as well as the autopsy results by Elliot and colleagues[13] support the hypothesis that surgery, after induction treatment, might improve local control and increase cure rates and survival.

Mixed Small Cell and Non–Small Cell Histology

A mixed SCLC–non-SCLC (NSCLC) histology was reported in 5% to 10% of surgical specimens.

Hirsch and colleagues[37] described 27 (7.2%) patients with small cell/large cell morphologic features in a series of 375 patients with SCLC. No difference in survival was observed between the different groups classified as oat cell and intermediate subtype, but a shorter survival was found in mixed histology patients (median 280 days vs 168 days). Other studies also demonstrated no clinically significant differences among the various histologic SCLC subtypes treated with CTx alone.[38,39] However, patients with mixed histology have a higher incidence of peripheral lesions on chest radiographs (56% vs 14%) but clinical characteristics similar to other SCLC subtypes. Patients with mixed SCLC treated with surgery and CTx survived more than 5 years.[40]

The University of Toronto Lung Oncology Group reported a series of 17 patients with mixed histology (14.3%) out of 119 patients with SCLC. Three patients with pretreatment had pure NSCLC at resection because of an excellent SCLC response to CTx with complete disappearance of the small cell component (**Table 1**).[41] From unpublished data from the author's clinic in Essen, among 260 patients with LD-SCLC treated with surgery and adjuvant CTx between 1985 and 2004, a mixed histology was found in 17 (6.9%). There were no significant differences between the 2 groups when surgical approach, perioperative outcome, and 5- and 10-year survival rates (37.5% and 23.0% for SCLC, 32.0% and 22.0% for mixed histology, respectively) were analyzed.

These findings suggest that the mixed subtype of SCLC is clinically comparable with pure SCLC as well as that surgery may play a central role in these specific tumors management. The possibility of a combined histology tumor should be considered in patients thought to have SCLC based on limited biopsy material, such as a

Table 1
Survival for patients with mixed SCLC and NSCLC histology

Author (Year)	Patients (N)	Survival
Carney et al,[38] 1980	8 of 103 (7.8%)	10.2 mo (only CTx)
Hirsch et al,[37] 1983	27 of 375 (7.2%)	168 d (only CTx)
Choi et al,[39] 1984	5 of 54 (9.0%)	—
Mangum et al,[40] 1989	9 of 429 (2.0%)	10 mo (2 patients >5 y after CTx/S)
Shepherd et al,[41] 1991	17 of 119 (14.3%)	111 wk (S/CTx or CTx/S)
(Stamatis, personal communication, 2004)	17 of 260 (6.9%)	32% and 22% after 5 y and 10 y

Abbreviation: S, surgery.

needle aspiration or bronchial biopsy, and when the primary lesion is peripheral.[41] In case of preoperative correct diagnosis, the initial treatment should be CTx in order to control the SCLC component; surgery should be considered to treat the CTx-resistant non–small cell component.

Salvage Operation for Initial Failure or Relapse

In patients with a poor response to CTx/chemoradiotherapy, or in patients with localized late relapse after the treatment of pure SCLCs, a repeated biopsy should be performed to rule out mixed NSCLC histopathology. The survival duration is extremely short after failure to respond or relapse after treatment, and second-line CTx or radiation has palliative intent only. Local control remains a problem, with one-third of patients with recurrences at the primary site. With the aim to prolong survival while achieving cure, the Toronto University Oncology Group undertook surgical resection in 28 patients with LD-SCLC who did not have complete remission with standard treatment or who had only local recurrence after treatment. The pathologic examination showed pure SCLC in 18 patients, mixed SCLC and NSCLC in 4, and pure NSCLC histology in 6. For the 10 mixed SCLC or NSCLC tumors, the median survival time after resection was greater than 2 years; 3 patients were alive 2 to 5 years after the diagnosis.[42] Yamada and colleagues[43] and Csekeo[44] published small series of selected patients with partial or absent response to CTx clinical. In the first one, 2 of 20 (10%) patients survived greater than 5 years, whereas, in the second, the 5-year survival rates were between 10% and 30% in patients with persistent N2 disease.

Synchronous Ipsilateral or Bilateral Small and Non–Small Cell Tumors

Because of the recent advanced techniques in imaging, the incidence of patients with synchronous ipsilateral or bilateral lung lesions is steadily increasing. Synchronous primary lung cancer occurs in up to 0.5% of patients with lung cancer. The coexistence of SCLC and NSCLC histology has been reported in a very small percentage by investigators from Japan.[45,46] A tumor has been first diagnosed intraoperatively or on pathologic examination of resected tissue in up to 40% of patients. Complete surgical resection was possible in more than 90% of cases, and CTx is usually administered.

Preoperative histologic diagnosis could be sometimes achieved through transbronchial biopsy or mediastinoscopy; induction CTx and surgical resection were performed.[47] Despite an early stage disease high frequency, surgical therapy yielded an overall 5-year survival between 20% and 36% only.[48] These findings suggest that the biology of such neoplasms is different from other primary lung cancers and that the second cancer might represent a metastatic disease.

A more accurate biologic definition of synchronous SCLCs and NSCLCs might be expected with the recent development of new molecular techniques, which include the analysis of DNA ploidy patterns or restriction fragment length polymorphism.

Second Primary Lung Cancer

Patients treated for SCLC are at a 7- to 16-fold-increased risk to develop a second primary tumor (SPT), mostly an NSCLC.[49] Up to 30% of patients who survive greater than 2 years after SCLC treatment will develop an SPT, and most are of aerodigestive origin.[50,51] Clinical series of second lung cancer (NSCLC and SCLC) have been published by several investigators.[52–54] Patients sometimes develop an NSCLC in the same lobe where the previous SCLC was located. Their treatment still represents a problem.[55] Additionally, metachronous malignancies can develop not only in the lung but also in other organs. Soria and colleagues[56] reviewed 1371 patients with SCLC with 8 metachronous malignancies between 1 and 6 years after the diagnosis of SCLC: of these,

3 were in the lung and 5 in other solid organs. Sagman and colleagues[53] have reported similar results.[53]

Most patients with SPT are treated with sublobar resection, whereas few receive lobectomy. This procedure is probably caused by the poor respiratory function as consequence of the previous intervention.

Smythe and colleagues[55] reported 29 patients with metachronous NSCLC: 11 received a surgical resection and 10 were at stage I. Squamous cell carcinoma was the most common histology. The median survival was 24.5 months, and the 5-year survival rate was 27%. The investigators concluded that surgical resection was feasible, but a poorer prognosis was evident, especially when compared with stage-matched control tumors.

An early stage SPT detection is usually the consequence of a strict clinical/radiological follow-up after SCLC treatment.

Johnson and colleagues[57] retrospectively analyzed 62 out of 578 patients who 2 years before were treated for SCLC: 20 patients developed a new SCLC and 15 an NSCLC.[57] The investigators recommended preventive CTx for long-term SCLC survivors.

Despite an early stage, SPT survival is poor; patients should be carefully selected for a possible surgical resection, and alternative treatment modalities (eg, stereotactic radiation) should also be taken into account.

PREOPERATIVE EVALUATION

Because of the SCLC's high risk of local and distant spread, a careful preoperative clinical/radiological evaluation is mandatory for patients potentially available for surgery.

Staging must include a thoracic and upper abdomen computed tomography scan, brain magnetic resonance imaging, and radionuclide bone scan. Bronchoscopy with endobronchial ultrasound and/or cervical mediastinoscopy or parasternal mediastinotomy for the left-sided tumors are necessary in case of suspicious mediastinal lymph-nodal involvement.

The use of an FDG-PET scan in the preoperative evaluation of patients with SCLC resulted in improvement on clinical staging as reported in small clinical series.[58–61]

Patients with SCLC should be evaluated in a multidisciplinary setting, which includes oncologists, radiation oncologists, pulmonologists, and surgeons; an overall risk-profile analysis is particularly important in case of restaging after induction treatment.

TREATMENT MODALITIES INCLUDING SURGERY
Surgery Alone

Today, the treatment of LD-SCLC with surgery alone has historical importance only. Merely old retrospective series indicate surgery alone for the treatment of stage I SCLC.[24,62]

Shore and Paneth[24] described 64 patients with bronchial oat cell carcinomas treated by surgery between 1959 and 1974: 24 of them underwent exploratory thoracotomy because of inoperable lesions. Of the 40 patients who underwent curative resection, only 11 were alive without recurrence. Ten of these survived 5 years or more, with an overall 5-year survival rate of 25%. In a retrospective study by Sorensen and colleagues,[25] 77 operated patients presented an SCLC. The TNM staging system was used to compare them with NSCLCs. Only 6 patients with T1-2, N0-1 disease survived, and 5- and 10-year survival rates were both 12%. CTx was not routinely used, and RTx was administered with palliative intent only.[25]

In the series by Maassen and colleagues[26] and Shah and colleagues,[63] better results of surgical treatment alone were observed: the investigators adopted an adequate preoperative staging, which also included mediastinoscopy; those patients with bulky disease were excluded (**Table 2**).

In the oldest series, sometimes bronchial carcinoids were falsely diagnosed as SCLC.

Surgery with Adjuvant CTx

At the end of the 1970s, systemic CTx with single or multiple regimes became the standard for either LD-SCLC or AD-SCLC treatment. The 2 combinations of cyclophosphamide, doxorubicin, and vincristine (CEV) and later cisplatin and etoposide (PE) seemed to be more effective and became widely used. In a randomized phase III trial, Sundstrøm and colleagues[64] investigated whether etoposide and cisplatin (PE) CTx was superior to CEV. The 2- and 5-year survival rates in the PE arm (14% and 5%) were significantly higher compared with those in the CEV one (6% and 2%). Among patients with LD-SCLC, the median survival time was 14.5 months versus 9.7 months, respectively.[65] Moreover, in patients with LD-SCLC, the PE combination became the preferred regimen because of its easy administration with concurrent thoracic radiotherapy.[66]

The VASOG trial in 1989 first demonstrated a survival improvement in 132 patients who received a potentially curative resection followed by an adjuvant CTx. The 5-year survival rates for each category were as follows: T1N0M0 59.9%, T1N1M0 31.3%, T2N0M0 27.9%, T2N1M0 9.0%, and any T3 or N2 3.6%. A 5-year survival rate of 80.8% was noted in those patients submitted to adjuvant CTx as compared with 38.1% in the group without CTx.[18] Many reports on surgery and adjuvant CTx date from the 1980s to early 2000. They are based on retrospective reviews with well-documented pathologic staging, so patients who received adjuvant treatment were more precisely staged compared with nonsurgical ones (**Table 3**).[18,67–88]

In stage I and II disease, the tumor was usually resected with a lobectomy (44%–72%), whereas pneumonectomy was the most common surgical procedure in stage III (48%–76%).

In many centers, postoperative CTx included 4 to 6 cycles (range: 1–18 cycles). In the latest publications from Cataldo, Suzuki, and Badzio,[82,83,85] the PE combination was largely used. Brock[89] reported different 5-year survival rates based on whether patients received platinum or nonplatinum CTx regimens (68.0% vs 32.2%).

No differences in survival were found between patients receiving 4 to 6 cycles compared with those treated longer; prolonged CTx has been, therefore, abandoned.[90]

Generally, the best survival rates were observed in patients with stage I disease (5-year rates between 26% and 76%), whereas the 5-year survival rates ranged from 14% to 50% and 0% to 40%, respectively, in stage II and III.[67–88] Survival was also longer in patients submitted to lobectomy

Table 2
Results of surgery alone in historical collectives (5-y survival by pathologicTNM stage)

Authors	Patients (N)	All Stages (%)	I (%)	II (%)	IIIa (%)
Shore & Paneth,[24] 1980	40	25.0	—	—	—
Li et al,[62] 1981	12	58.3[a]	—	—	—
Maaßen et al,[26] 1985	66	17.0	40.0	9.0	14.0
Sørensen et al,[25] 1986	77	8.0	12.0	13.0	0
Shah et al,[63] 1992	28	43.3	57.1	—	55.5

[a] Greater than 2 years.

Table 3
Results of surgery and adjuvant CTx (5-y survival by pathologicTNM stage)

Author	Patients (N)	CTx	Total (%)	Stage I (%)	Stage II (%)	Stage III (%)
Hayata et al,[67] 1978	72	CAV	11	26	17	0
Shields et al,[18] 1982	132	CAV	31	48	24	24
Meyer et al,[68,69] 1983, 1984	30	—	—	50	50	0
Ohta et al,[70] 1986	24	Various	30.7	50.8	0	0
Osterlind et al,[71] 1986	36	—	—	22	28	—
Maassen et al,[26] 1985	124	CAV	20 (3 y)	34	21	11
Shepherd et al,[73] 1988	63	Various	31	48	24	24
Karrer et al,[74] 1989	112	CAV	—	62 (3 y)	50 (3 y)	41 (3 y)
Macchiarini et al,[75] 1991	42	—	36	52	—	13
Hara et al,[76] 1991	37	Various	32	64	42	11
Davis et al,[77] 1993	37	CAV	26	50	35	21
Karrer & Ulsperger,[78] 1995	157	CAV	—	56	29	33
Lucchi et al,[79] 1997	92	CAV	32.5	45.7	14.6	9.0
Rea et al,[80] 1998	104	CAV	32.0	52.2	30.0	15.3
Shepherd,[81] 2000	63	Various	31	48	24	24
Cataldo,[82] 2000	60	CAV, PE	—	40	36	15
Suzuki et al,[83] 2000	62	PE	57	76	38	40
Kobayashi et al,[84] 2000	59	Various	—	55	33	23
Badzio et al,[85] 2001	67	—	27	—	—	—
(Stamatis, personal communication, 2004)	260	CAV, PE	37.5	42.0	28.6	15.6
Wang et al,[86] 2007	122	Various	38.0	57.1	43.9	28.3
Ju et al,[87] 2012	34	PE	66.4 (3 y)	84.0 (3 y)		13.0 (3 y)
Ogawa et al,[88] 2012	19	PE	47	—	—	—

Abbreviation: CAV, c for cyclophosphamide, a for doxorubicin and v for vincristine.

rather than limited resection (50% vs 20%).[89] Lucchi[79] described 47.2%, 14.8%, and 14.4% survival rates for stage I, II, and III, respectively. Patients with N0 lesions had a significantly better outcome than patients with N1 and N2 lesions.[79] The University of Toronto Lung Oncology Group published similar results.[81]

Tsuchiya and colleagues[90] reported the prospective phase II trial results on adjuvant treatment with PE after the initial complete resection in stage I to IIIA SCLCs. Ninety-seven percent of patients had a complete mediastinal node dissection. The overall relapse rate was 10%; it was 6% in stage I but 22% in stage IIIa disease.[90] The cumulative incidence of recurrence (distant) was 26%, with the brain as the most common (15% of cases). PCI was then recommended after adjuvant CTx in patients with good performance status who underwent a complete resection.[90,91]

The inclusion of CTx as adjuvant treatment seems to improve survival compared with surgery alone.

Induction CTx Followed by Surgery

Even in recent CTx protocols, most patients with SCLC experience recurrences or distant metastases. Studies revealed a vital residual disease rate at the primary site between 55% and 80% at autopsy or after adjuvant surgery.[13,41]

Concerning the encouraging results with primary surgery followed by adjuvant CTx, several investigators started prospective studies with induction CTx in LD-NSCLC.

Arguments for this treatment preference were as follows: (1) patients' better general condition before surgery, making them suitable for a complete CTx administration, and (2) the CTx downstaging effect with potential distant metastasis reduction. Retrospective analysis and nonrandomized trials are summarized in **Table 4**.

Different CTx regimens have been used, mostly CAV or PE.[15,92–102] The response rates ranged between 50% and 100% after the administration

Table 4
Results of neoadjuvant CTx followed by surgery (5-y survival by pathologicTNM stage)

Investigator	N	Protocol	Total (%)	Med Surv (mo)	pStage I	pStage II (%)	pStage III (%)
Prager et al,[92] 1984	39	CAV	—	17/11	—	—	—
Williams et al,[93] 1987	38	CAE	—	33	—	—	—
Johnson et al,[94] 1987	24	CAV, PE	—	—	—	—	—
Baker et al,[95] 1987	37	CA, E	—	—	—	—	—
Shepherd et al,[15] 1989	76	CAV, PE	36	21	70%	35	20
Benfield et al,[111] 1989	8	CAV, E	—	—	—	—	—
Hara et al,[96] 1991	17	Various	33	—	MS 26 mo	100	0
Zatopek et al,[97] 1991	25	Various	—	—	—	—	—
Wada et al,[98] 1995	17	Various	31	—	80%	—	10
Fujimori et al,[99] 1997	21	CAV	29	61.9	—	—	—
Lewiński et al,[100] 2001	35	E-based	29	18.5	44%	12	—
Nakamura et al,[101] 2004	37	Various	—	—	48.9%	33.3	20.2
Veronesi et al,[102] 2007	23	Car/VP16	—	24	—	—	—

Abbreviations: CAE, c for cyclophosphamide, a for doxorubicin and e for etoposide; Car/VP16, carboplatin/etoposide (for etoposide there are two abbreviations, E or VP16); CAV, c for Cyclophosphamide, a for doxorubicin and v for vincristine; Med Surv, median survival; MS, median survival (like Med Surv); pStage, pathologic stage.

of 2 and 6 CTx cycles,[17] and the reported perioperative morbidity and mortality was not higher than those observed when surgery was followed by adjuvant CTx. The complete surgical resection (R0) rate varied between 65% and 100%. Nevertheless, the number of patients who underwent surgical exploration was small in many series.

There are controversial reports about surgery after induction CTx. In a recent report, Yuequan and colleagues[103] retrospectively analyzed the survival rates after lobectomy and pneumonectomy for patients with stage II and III SCLC. Out of 75 patients, 31 underwent pneumonectomy and 44 lobectomy. The overall survival rate after pneumonectomy was significantly better compared with that after lobectomy in patients with stage II tumors, but no difference was found between the 2 groups in patients with stage III tumors. The local recurrence rate after lobectomy was higher than in the pneumonectomy group.[103] In the report of Yu and colleagues[21] from 1560 patients with SCLC, 121 (7.8%) had a sublobar resection, 247 (15.8%) a lobectomy, 10 (0.6%) a pneumonectomy, and 21 an unspecified surgical procedure (1.35%); the remaining 1161 patients did not received an operation. The 5-year overall survival rates in the overall cohort of patients was 21.1%; it was 50.3% after lobectomy, 45.7% after pneumonectomy, and 33.7% after sublobar resection.[21] Weksler and colleagues[20] evaluated, in another SEER report, the outcome of 3566 patients with stage I and II SCLC between 1988 and 2007. Surgical treatment was performed in 895

(25.1%); among them, a wedge resection was done in 251 (28.0%) and lobectomy or pneumonectomy in 637 (71.2%). The median survival after lobectomy/pneumonectomy was 39 months; it was significantly longer than after wedge resection (28 months), which was higher than the median survival of not-operated patients (16 months).[20]

Although in older series the number of pneumonectomies was relatively high compared with lobectomies, published reports after 1990 showed a significant trend to resect SCLC tumors mainly by lobectomy avoiding pneumonectomy.[21,87,103] Sleeve resections are rarely described because the radicality of these procedures in patients with SCLC is not well defined.[104,105]

The lymph-nodal staging remains an important prognostic factor, not least to properly allocate patients in a true pathologic stage.[20] In a retrospective review of 104 patients with SCLC, Riquet and colleagues[106] performed 51 lobectomies and 53 pneumonectomies. The postoperative mortality was 5.7%, and the 5-year survival rate depended strongly on stage: 34.3% in stage I, 26.2% in stage II, and 2.7% in stage III. There were no 5-year survivors among patients with N2 lesions.[106] Granetzky and colleagues[107] reported a significant improvement of survival in patients with complete histologic tumor regression in the mediastinal lymph nodes after induction treatment (31.7 months) compared with those with persistent mediastinal lymph nodal involvement detected after thoracotomy (12.4 months).[107]

Lewinski and colleagues[100] pointed out that no residual tumor in the resected specimen Pathologic complete response (pCR) was the most favorable prognostic factor, and they also proposed to not perform surgery in case of persistent N2 disease.[100] Hanagiri and colleagues[108] found that, in stages II and IIIA, only those patients who respond to induction CTx may have a chance to survive after surgery. In stage II and IIIA, only CTx responders with a completely resectable tumor had a median survival time of 46 months and 3- and 5-year survival of 57.2% and 38.3%, respectively.[108]

Wada and colleagues[98] observed how the 5-year survival rate of patients with c-stage III SCLC in the neoadjuvant group, although not satisfactory (10.0%), was significantly higher compared with the adjuvant therapy (0.0%, $P = .04$). Considering the advantage of preoperative CTx and the discrepancy between c and p stage, sufficient intensity of combination CTx before surgery should be used and may result in a good prognosis for patients with c-stage I or II disease. In contrast, patients with c-stage III disease are not appropriate candidates for surgery even if preoperative CTx is performed.[98]

Many series comprised a small number of patients, whereas some investigators also included patients treated with salvage operations.

Induction Chemoradiotherapy Followed by Surgery

Two studies reported the use of induction chemoradiotherapy followed by surgery for LD-SCLC. The first reported a retrospective study with induction CTx and concurrent split course thoracic radiotherapy followed by surgery in patients having an objective response. The median survival time for all patients was 16 months, with 12.1% of the long-term survivors still living after 2 years and 9% living after 3 and 4 years.[109] This study showed a high CTx efficacy; but unfortunately, the number of patients who finally underwent surgery was too small to draw any meaningful conclusions.

The second study was a prospective phase II trial with platinum-based induction CTx, followed by RTx-CTx and definitive surgery, reported by Eberhardt and colleagues[110] from the Essen group. Following mediastinoscopy, a prognostically orientated aggressive approach was chosen in selected patients. Patients with stage IB/IIA disease had 4 PE cycles followed by surgery. Patients with stage IIB/IIIA disease had 3 PE cycles followed by one cycle of concurrent RTx-CTx including hyperfractionated accelerated radiation and then surgery. Most patients with stage IIIB disease were not planned for surgery and had CTx followed by sequential radiotherapy or one cycle of concurrent RTx-CTx. Of 46 consecutive patients (stage IB: 6, IIA: 2, IIB/IIIA: 22, IIIB: 16), 43 (94%) showed an objective response. Routinely, PCI (30-Gy in 3 weeks in daily 2-Gy fractions) was started after the end of the fourth CTx cycle on day 9 of thoracic irradiation in patients with RTx-CTx or was given after the thoracotomy in patients with stages IB/IIA. Only patients with negative mediastinal nodes by repeat mediastinoscopy after the induction treatment were considered for surgery. Twenty-three patients (72%) were completely resected (R0) (stage IB: 6 of 6, IIA: 2 of 2, IIB/IIIA: 13 of 22, IIIB: 2 of 2). Surgical procedures were as follows: pneumonectomy (10 cases), bilobectomy (2), and lobectomy (11). The overall toxicity was acceptable (1 patient died of septicemia), and no perioperative deaths occurred. The overall median survival and 5-year survival rates were 36 months and 46%, respectively, and 68 months and 63% in patients with R0 tumors. Of the 23 completely resected SCLC, 12 (52%) had viable tumor tissue. Histologic examination revealed 9 patients with vital pure small cell carcinoma and 3 with NSCLC (2 squamous cell and 1 large cell anaplastic carcinoma). The remaining 11 patients had no vital tumor in the resected specimens. No patients with N0 at repeat mediastinoscopy had microscopic N2 status in the final pathology. Of the 23 patients with R0 tumors, 9 (36%) developed relapses (8 isolated central nervous system and 1 liver). The Essen study showed that, in highly selected patients with stage IIB/IIIA disease, an aggressive multimodality treatment was feasible with acceptable toxicities and resulted in highly effective local control and remarkable long-term survival.

SUMMARY

Although 2 randomized trials of limited SCLC have failed to show any benefit from the addition of surgery to the multimodality treatment, retrospective analysis and prospective nonrandomized studies suggest that surgical resection, if a part of a multimodal treatment of stage I and II SCLC, is associated with significant improvement of local control and disease-free survival. Neoadjuvant CTx followed by surgery was feasible with controllable toxicities and acceptable perioperative morbidity and mortality rates.

In patients with SCLC, the IASLC and the American Joint Committee on Cancer/International Union Against Cancer recommend the use of the seventh edition of the TNM staging system to classify tumor stage. Stratification should be incorporated in clinical trials of early stage disease. The operability criteria adopted in patients with NSCLC are probably also appropriate for SCLC.

In patients with clinical LD-SCLC, PET imaging is recommended as well as an invasive mediastinal staging and extrathoracic imaging.

The following groups of patients could potentially benefit from surgical resection:

1. Patients with small lesion unexpectedly identified as SCLC at the time of thoracotomy. Complete resection and systematic lymph node dissection should be undertaken. CTx is recommended postoperatively, and PCI should also be considered.
2. In stage I and II SCLC after CTx and tumor response, surgery can improve local control and increase cure rates and long-term survival. Complete resection and mediastinal lymph node resection should be performed. In case of tumors with mixed histology, an initial CTx should control the SCLC growth; subsequently, surgery might resect the NSCLC component.
3. In patients with initial CTx failure or those with localized late relapse after completed treatment of pure SCLC, a salvage operation may be considered on an individual basis.
4. In patients with a second primary SCLC or NSCLC after a cured SCLC, surgery should be considered in the course of a multidisciplinary approach.
5. Patients with synchronous ipsilateral or bilateral SCLC and NSCLC could be potential candidates for surgery in a diagnostic or therapeutic intention.
6. In selected patients with IIIA N2 disease and complete histologic regression of tumor tissue in the mediastinal lymph nodes after induction CTx or CTx-RTx, surgery can improve local control and survival.

Finally, to improve the current management strategies for SCLC, surgeons should participate in patients' assessment together with oncologists and radiotherapists and common guidelines for indications and therapy concepts should be adopted. Interdisciplinary approaches should be also used in controlled clinical trials.

REFERENCES

1. Devesa SS, Bray F, Vizcaino AP, et al. International lung cancer trends by histologic type: male:female differences diminishing and adenocarcinoma rates rising. Int J Cancer 2005;117:294–9.
2. Rostad H, Naalsund A, Jacobsen R, et al. Small cell lung cancer in Norway. Should more patients have been offered surgical therapy? Eur J Cardiothorac Surg 2004;26:782–6.
3. Hansen HH, Dombernowsky P, Hirsch FR. Staging procedures and prognostic features in small cell lung anaplastic carcinoma. Semin Oncol 1978;5:280–7.
4. Zelen M. Keynote address on biostatic data retrieval. Cancer Chemother Rep 3 1973;4:31–42.
5. Travis WD, Colby TV, Corrin B, et al. Histologic typing of lung and pleural tumors. In: World Health Organization international classification of tumors. Berlin: Springen; 1999. p. 7–12.
6. Shepherd FA, Crowley J, Van Houte P, et al, International Association for the Study of Lung Cancer International Staging Committee and Participating Institutions. The International Association for the Study of Lung Cancer lung cancer staging project: proposals regarding the clinical staging of small cell lung cancer in the forthcoming (seventh) edition of the tumor, node, metastasis classification for lung cancer. J Thorac Oncol 2007;2:1067–77.
7. Valliéres E, Shepherd FA, Crowley J, et al, International Association for the Study of Lung Cancer International Staging Committee and Participating Institutions. The IASLC Lung Cancer Staging Project: proposals regarding the relevance of TNM in the pathological staging of small cell lung cancer in the forthcoming (seventh) edition of the TNM classification for lung cancer. J Thorac Oncol 2009;4:1049–59.
8. Goldman KP. Histology of lung cancer in relation to prognosis. Thorax 1965;20:298–302.
9. Lennox SC, Flavell G, Pollock DJ, et al. Results of resection for oat cell carcinoma of the lung. Lancet 1968;2:925–7.
10. Fox W, Scadding JG. Medical Research Council comparative trial of surgery and radiotherapy for primary treatment of small-celled or oat-celled carcinoma of the bronchus. Ten-year follow-up. Lancet 1973;2(7820):63–5.
11. Szczesny TJ, Szczesna A, Shepherd FA, et al. Surgical treatment of small cell lung cancer. Semin Oncol 2003;30:47–56.
12. Livinston RB. Current CT of small cell lung cancer. Chest 1986;89:2585–635.
13. Elliott SA, Osterlind K, Hirsch FR, et al. Metastatic patterns in small-cell lung cancer: correlation of autopsy findings and clinical parameters in 537 patients. J Clin Oncol 1987;5:246–54.
14. Arriagada R, Le Chevalier T, Borie F, et al. Prophylactic cranial irradiation for patients with small cell lung cancer in complete remission. J Natl Cancer Inst 1995;87:183–90.
15. Shepherd FA, Ginsberg RJ, Patterson GA, et al. A prospective study of adjuvant surgical resection

after CT for limited small cell lung cancer. J Thorac Cardiovasc Surg 1989;97:177–86.

16. Lad T, Piantadosi S, Thomas P, et al. A prospective randomized trial to determine the benefit of surgical resection of residual disease following response of small cell lung cancer to combination CT. Chest 1994;106:320–3.

17. Waddell TK, Shepherd FA. Should aggressive surgery ever be part of the management of small cell lung cancer? Thorac Surg Clin 2004;14:271–81.

18. Shields TW, Higgins GA Jr, Matthews MJ, et al. Surgical resection in the management of small cell lung carcinoma of the lung. J Thorac Cardiovasc Surg 1982;84:481–8.

19. Shields TW. Surgery of small cell lung cancer. Chest 1986;89:264S–7S.

20. Weksler B, Nason KS, Shende M, et al. Surgical resection should be considered for stage I and II small cell carcinoma of the lung. Ann Thorac Surg 2012;94:889–93.

21. Yu JB, Decker RH, Detterbeck FC, et al. Surveillance Epidemiology and End Results evaluation on the role of surgery for stage I small cell lung cancer. J Thorac Oncol 2010;5:215–9.

22. Califano R, Abidin AZ, Peck R, et al. Management of small cell lung cancer: recent developments for optimal care. Drugs 2012;72:471–90.

23. Ferraldeschi R, Baka S, Jyoti B, et al. Modern management of small cell lung cancer. Drugs 2007;67:2135–52.

24. Shore DF, Paneth M. Survival after resection of small cell carcinoma of the bronchus. Thorax 1980;35:819–22.

25. Sørensen HR, Lund C, Alstrup P. Survival in small cell lung carcinoma after surgery. Thorax 1986;41:479–82.

26. Maassen W, Greschuchna D, Martinez I. The role of surgery in the treatment of small cell carcinoma of the lung. In: Recent results in cancer research, vol. 97. Berlin (Germany): Springer Verlag Berlin-Heidelberg; 1985. p. 107–15.

27. Jett JR, Schild SE, Kesler KA, et al. Treatment of small cell lung cancer. Diagnosis and management of lung cancer, 3rd ed: American College of Chest Physicians evidence-based clinical practice guidelines. Chest 2013;143:400S–19S.

28. Idhe DC, Pass HI, Glatstein EJ. Small cell lung cancer. In: DeVita VT Jr, Hellmann S, Rosenberg SA, editors. Cancer: principles and practice of oncology. 5th edition. Philadelphia:: Lippincott; 1985. p. 911–49.

29. Pignon JP, Arriagada R, Idhe DC, et al. A meta-analysis of thoracic radiotherapy for small cell lung cancer. N Engl J Med 1992;327:1618–24.

30. Elias AD. Small cell lung cancer: state of the art therapy in 1996. Chest 1997;112:251S–8S.

31. Gray JR, Sobczak ML, Hahn SM, et al. Analysis of local control in 150 limited stage small cell lung cancer patients treated with combined thoracic irradiation and multiagent CT. Proc Am Soc Clin Oncol 1995;14:349 [abstract 1056].

32. Souhami RL, Law K. Longevity in small cell lung cancer. A report to the Lung Cancer Subcommittee of the United Kingdom Coordinating Committee for Cancer Research. Br J Cancer 1990;61:584–9.

33. Thomas CR Jr, Giroux DJ, Janaki LM, et al. Ten-year follow-up of Southwest Oncology Group 8269: a phase II trial of concomitant cisplatin-etoposide and daily thoracic radiotherapy in limited small cell lung cancer. Lung Cancer 2001;33:213–9.

34. Warde P, Payne D. Does thoracic irradiation improve survival and local control in limited-stage small-cell carcinoma of the lung? A meta-analysis. J Clin Oncol 1992;10:890–5.

35. Turrisi AT, Kim K, Blum R, et al. Twice-daily compared with once-daily thoracic radiotherapy in limited small-cell lung cancer treated concurrently with cisplatin and etoposide. N Engl J Med 1999;340:265–71.

36. Schreiber D, Rineer J, Weedon J, et al. Survival outcomes with the use of surgery in limited-stage small cell lung cancer. Cancer 2010;116:1350–7.

37. Hirsch FR, Osterlind K, Hansen HH. The prognosis significance of histopathologic subtyping of small cell carcinoma of the lung according to the classification of the World Health Organization. A study of 375 consecutive patients. Cancer 1983;52:2144–50.

38. Carney DN, Matthews MJ, Ihde DC, et al. Influence of histologic subtype of small cell carcinoma of the lung on clinical presentation, response to therapy, and survival. J Natl Cancer Inst 1980;65:1225–30.

39. Choi H, Byhardt RW, Clowry LJ, et al. The prognostic significance of histologic subtyping in small cell carcinoma of the lung. Am J Clin Oncol 1984;7:389–97.

40. Mangum MD, Greco FA, Hainsworth JD, et al. Combined small cell and non-small-cell lung cancer. J Clin Oncol 1989;7:607–12.

41. Shepherd FA, Ginsberg RJ, Feld R, et al. Surgical treatment for limited small cell lung cancer. The University of Toronto Lung Oncology Group experience. J Thorac Cardiovasc Surg 1991;101:385–93.

42. Shepherd FA, Ginsberg R, Patterson GA, et al. Is there ever a role for salvage operations in limited small-cell lung cancer? J Thorac Cardiovasc Surg 1991;101:196–200.

43. Yamada K, Saijo N, Kojima A, et al. A retrospective analysis of patients receiving surgery after CT for small cell lung cancer. Jpn J Clin Oncol 1991;21:39–45.

44. Csekeo A. The possibility of surgery for small cell lung cancer (state of the art). Magy Onkol 2006;50:223–7.

45. Niho S, Yokose T, Nagai K, et al. A case of synchronous double primary lung cancer with neuroendocrine features. Jpn J Clin Oncol 1999;29(4):219–25.

46. Nishiyama H, Kaguraoka H, Kuroki M, et al. Multiple primary cancers in surgically resected lung cancer patients. Nihon Kyobu Geka Gakkai Zasshi 1989;37:56–61.

47. Hiraki A, Ueoka H, Yoshino T, et al. Synchronous primary lung cancer presenting with small cell carcinoma and non-small cell carcinoma: diagnosis and treatment. Oncol Rep 1999;6:75–80.

48. Kondo K, Monden Y. Therapy for multiple primary lung cancers. Kyobu Geka 2002;55:4–9.

49. Johnson BE, Contazar P, Chute JP. Second lung cancers in patients successfully treated for lung cancer. Semin Oncol 1997;24:492–9.

50. Heyne KH, Lippmann SM, Lee JJ, et al. The incidence of second primary tumors in long-term survivors of small-cell lung cancer. J Clin Oncol 1992; 10:1519–24.

51. Kawahara M, Ushijima S, Kamimori T, et al. Second primary tumors in more than 2 year disease free survivors of small-cell lung cancer in Japan: the role of smoking cessation. Br J Cancer 1998;78: 409–12.

52. Reinmuth N, Stumpf A, Stumpf P, et al. Characteristics and outcome of patients with second primary lung cancer [abstract]. Eur Respir J 2012;42(6): 1668–76.

53. Sagman U, Lishner M, Maki E, et al. Second primary malignancies following diagnosis of small-call lung cancer. J Clin Oncol 1992;10:1525–33.

54. Szczepek B, Szymanska D, Decker E, et al. Risk of late recurrence and/or second lung cancer after treatment of patients with small cell lung cancer (SCLC). Lung Cancer 1994;11:93–104.

55. Smythe WR, Estrera AL, Swisher SG, et al. Surgical resection of non-small cell carcinoma after treatment of small cell carcinoma. Ann Thorac Surg 2001;71:962–6.

56. Soria JC, Bréchot JM, Lebeau B, et al. Second primary cancers after small-cell lung cancer. Bull Cancer 1997;84:800–6.

57. Johnson BE, Linnolla RI, Williams JP, et al. Risk of second aerodigestive cancers increases in patients who survive free of small cell lung cancer for more than 2 years. J Clin Oncol 1995;13:101–11.

58. Schumacher T, Brink I, Mix M, et al. FDG-PET imaging for the staging and follow-up of small cell lung cancer. Eur J Nucl Med 2001;28:483–8.

59. Zhao DS, Valdivia AY, Li Y, et al. 18F-fluorodeoxyglucose positron emission tomography in small-cell lung cancer. Semin Nucl Med 2002;32:272–5.

60. Kamel EM, Zwahlen D, Wyss MT, et al. Whole-body (18)F-FDG PET improves the management of patients with small cell lung cancer. J Nucl Med 2003;44:1911–7.

61. Bradley JD, Dehdashti F, Mintun MA, et al. Positron emission tomography in limited-stage small-cell lung cancer: a prospective study. Clin Oncol 2004;22(16):3248–54.

62. Li W, Hammar SP, Jolly PC, et al. Unpredictable course of small cell undifferentiated lung carcinoma. J Thorac Cardiovasc Surg 1981;81:34–43.

63. Shah SS, Thompson J, Goldstraw P. Results of operation without adjuvant therapy in the treatment of small cell lung cancer. Ann Thorac Surg 1992; 54:498–501.

64. Sundstrøm S, Bremnes RM, Kaasa S, et al. Cisplatin and etoposide regimen is superior to cyclophosphamide, epirubicin, and vincristine regimen in small-cell lung cancer: results from a randomized phase III trial with 5 years' follow-up. J Clin Oncol 2002;20:4665–72.

65. Laurie SA, Logan D, Markman BR, et al. Practice guideline for the role of combination CT in the initial management of limited-stage small-cell lung cancer. Lung Cancer 2004;43:223–40.

66. McCracken JD, Janaki LM, Crowley JJ, et al. Concurrent CT/radiotherapy for limited small-cell lung carcinoma: a Southwest Oncology Group Study. J Clin Oncol 1990;8:892–8.

67. Hayata Y, Funatsu H, Suemasu K, et al. Surgical indications for small cell carcinoma of the lung. Jpn J Clin Oncol 1978;8:93–100.

68. Meyer JA, Comis RL, Ginsberg SJ, et al. The prospect of disease control by surgery combined with CT in stage I and stage II small cell carcinoma of the lung. Ann Thorac Surg 1983;36:37–41.

69. Meyer JA, Gullo JJ, Ikins PM, et al. Adverse prognostic effect of N2 disease in treated small cell carcinoma of the lung. J Thorac Cardiovasc Surg 1984;88:495–501.

70. Ohta M, Hara N, Ichinose Y, et al. The role of surgical resection in the management of small cell carcinoma of the lung. Jpn J Clin Oncol 1986;16:289–96.

71. Osterlind K, Hansen M, Hansen HH, et al. Influence of surgical resection prior to CT on the long-term results in small cell lung cancer. A study of 250 operable patients. Eur J Cancer Clin Oncol 1986;22: 589–93.

72. Maassen W, Greschuchna D. Small cell carcinoma of the lung–to operate or not? Surgical experience and results. Thorac Cardiovasc Surg 1986;34:71–6.

73. Shepherd FA, Evans WK, Feld R, et al. Adjuvant CT following surgical resection for small-cell carcinoma of the lung. J Clin Oncol 1988;6:832–8.

74. Karrer K, Denck H, Karnicka-Mlodkowska H, et al. The role of ifosfamide and cyclophosphamide in the multi-modality treatment after surgery for cure for small-cell bronchial carcinomas (SCLC). Med Oncol Tumor Pharmacother 1989;6:143–9.

75. Macchiarini P, Hardin M, Basolo F, et al. Surgery plus adjuvant CT for T1-3N0M0 small-cell lung

cancer. Rationale for current approach. Am J Clin Oncol 1991;14:218–24.

76. Hara N, Ichinose Y, Kuda T, et al. Long-term survivors in resected and nonresected small cell lung cancer. Oncology 1991;48:441–7.

77. Davis S, Crino L, Tonato M, et al. A prospective analysis of CT following surgical resection of clinical stage I-II small-cell lung cancer. Am J Clin Oncol 1993;16:93–5.

78. Karrer K, Ulsperger E. Surgery for cure followed by CT in small cell carcinoma of the lung. For the ISC-Lung Cancer Study Group. Acta Oncol 1995;34: 899–906.

79. Lucchi M, Mussi A, Chella A, et al. Surgery in the management of small cell lung cancer. Eur J Cardiothorac Surg 1997;12(5):689–93.

80. Rea F, Callegaro D, favaretto A, et al. Long term results of surgery and CT in small cell lung cancer. Eur J Cardiothorac Surg 1998;14:398–402.

81. Shepherd FA. Surgical management of small-cell lung cancer. In: Pass HI, Mitchell JB, Johnson DH, et al, editors. Lung cancer: principles and practice. Baltimore (MD): Lippincott Williams & Wilkins; 2000. p. 889–913. Philadelphia: Raven; p. 967–80.

82. Cataldo I. Long term survival for resectable small cell lung cancer. Lung Cancer 2000;29:130–2.

83. Suzuki R, Tsuchiya R, Ichinose Y, et al. Phase II trial of post-operative adjuvant cisplatin/etoposide (PE) in patients with completely resected SCLC. Proc Am Soc Clin Oncol 2000;19:492a [abstract 1925].

84. Kobayashi S, Okada S, Hasumi T, et al. Combined modality therapy including surgery for stage III stage III small cell lung cancer on the basis of the sensitivity assay in vitro. Surg Today 2000;30: 127–33.

85. Badzio A, Jassern J, Kurowski K, et al. The role of surgery in limited disease (LD) small cell lung cancer (SCLC): retrospective comparative study. Eur J Cancer 2001;37:61.

86. Wang HJ, Sun KL, Zhang XR, et al. Combined modality therapy for small cell lung cancer patient with limited stage disease. Zhonghua Zhong Liu Za Zhi 2007;29:701–9.

87. Ju MH, Kim HR, Kim JB, et al. Surgical outcomes in small cell lung cancer. Korean J Thorac Cardiovasc Surg 2012;45:40–4.

88. Ogawa S, Horio Y, Yatabe Y, et al. Patterns of recurrence and outcome in patients with surgically resected small cell lung cancer. Int J Clin Oncol 2012;17:218–24.

89. Brock MV, Hooker CM, Syphard JE, et al. Surgical resection of limited disease small cell lung cancer in the new era of platinum CT: its time has come. J Thorac Cardiovasc Surg 2005;129:64–72.

90. Tsuchiya R, Suzuki K, Ichinose Y, et al. Phase II trial of postoperative adjuvant cisplatin and etoposide in patients with completely resected stage I-IIIa

small cell lung cancer: the Japan Clinical Oncology Lung Cancer Study Group Trial (JCOG9101). J Thorac Cardiovasc Surg 2005;129:977–83.

91. Bischof M, Debus J, Herfarth K, et al. Surgery and CT for small cell lung cancer in stage I-II with or without radiotherapy. Strahlenther Onkol 2007;183: 679–84.

92. Prager RL, Foster JM, Hainsworth JD, et al. The feasibility of adjuvant surgery in limited-stage small cell carcinoma: a prospective evaluation. Ann Thorac Surg 1984;38(6):622–6.

93. Williams CJ, McMillan I, Lea R, et al. Surgery after initial CT for localized small-cell carcinoma of the lung. J Clin Oncol 1987;5(10):1579–88.

94. Johnson DH, Einhorn LH, Mandelbaum I, et al. Post CT resection of residual tumor in limited stage small cell lung cancer. Chest 1987;92(2):241–6.

95. Baker RR, Ettinger DS, Ruckdeschel JD, et al. The role of surgery in the management of selected patients with small-cell carcinoma of the lung. Oncol 1987;5(5):697–702.

96. Hara N, Ohta M, Ichinose Y, et al. Influence of surgical resection before and after CT on survival in small cell lung cancer. J Surg Oncol 1991;47(1):53–61.

97. Zatopek NK, Holoye PY, Ellerbroek NA, et al. Resectability of small-cell lung cancer following induction CT in patients with limited disease (stage II-IIIb). Am J Clin Oncol 1991;14(5):427–32.

98. Wada H, Yokomise H, Tanaka F, et al. Surgical treatment of small cell carcinoma of the lung: advantage of preoperative CT. Lung Cancer 1995;13(1):45–56.

99. Fujimori K, Yokoyama A, Kurita Y, et al. A pilot phase 2 study of surgical treatment after induction CT for resectable stage I to IIIA small cell lung cancer. Chest 1997;11:1089–93.

100. Lewiński T, Zuławski M, Turski C, et al. Small cell lung cancer I–III A: cytoreductive CT followed by resection with continuation of CT. Eur J Cardiothorac Surg 2001;20(2):391–8.

101. Nakamura H, Kato Y, Kato H. Outcome of surgery for small cell lung cancer. Response to induction CT predicts survival. Thorac Cardiovasc Surg 2004;52:206–10.

102. Veronesi G, scanagatta P, Leo F, et al. Adjuvant surgery after carboplatin and VP16 in resectable small cell lung cancer. J Thorac Oncol 2007;2:131–4.

103. Yuequan J, Zhi Z, Chenmin X. Surgical resection for small cell lung cancer: pneumonectomy versus lobectomy [abstract]. ISRN Surg 2012;2012: 101024.

104. Veronesi G, Solli PG, Leo F, et al. Low morbidity of bronchoplastic procedures after CT for lung cancer. Lung Cancer 2002;36:91–7.

105. Leo F, Pastorino U. Surgery in small cell lung carcinoma. Where is the rationale? Semin Surg Oncol 2003;21:176–81.

106. Riquet M, Le Pimpec Barthes F, Scotté F, et al. Relevance of surgery in small cell lung cancer. Rev Pneumol Clin 2009;65:129–35.

107. Granetzny A, Boseila A, Wagner W, et al. Surgery in the tri-modality treatment of small cell lung cancer. Stage-dependent survival. Eur J Cardiothorac Surg 2006;30(2):212–6.

108. Hanagiri T, Sugio K, Baba T, et al. Results of surgical treatment for patients with small cell lung cancer. J Thorac Oncol 2009;4:964–8.

109. Gridelli C, D'Aprile M, Curcio C, et al. Carboplatin plus epirubicin plus VP-16, concurrent 'split course' radiotherapy and adjuvant surgery for limited small cell lung cancer. Gruppo Oncologico Centro-Sud-Isole (GOCSI). Lung Cancer 1994;11:83–91.

110. Eberhardt W, Stamatis G, Stuschke M, et al. Prognostically orientated multimodality treatment including surgery for selected patients of small-cell lung cancer patients stage Ib to IIIB: long-term results of a phase II trial. Br J Cancer 1999;81:1206–12.

111. Benfield GF, Matthews HR, Watson DC, et al. Chemotherapy plus adjuvant surgery for local small cell lung cancer. Eu J Surg Oncol 1989;15:341–5.

Thymic Neuroendocrine Tumors

Paolo Olivo Lausi, MD[a], Majed Refai, MD[b], Pier Luigi Filosso, MD[a], Enrico Ruffini, MD[a], Alberto Oliaro, MD[a], Francesco Guerrera, MD[a], Alessandro Brunelli, MD[c,]*

KEYWORDS

- Thymus • Neuroendocrine tumors • Surgery • Chemotherapy • Radiotherapy • Outcome

KEY POINTS

- Thymic neuroendocrine tumors are rare and account for approximately 2% to 5% of all thymic tumors.
- Despite the suggestion of benign behavior implied by their name, thymic carcinoids have been noted to present a more aggressive biologic behavior than their counterparts in other sites.
- Because of the lack of data, adequate-sized prospective trials are required for validation and the enrollment of patients with advanced disease into available clinical trials is encouraged.

EPIDEMIOLOGY

Thymic neuroendocrine tumors (NETs) are rare and account for approximately 2% to 5% of all thymic tumors.[1,2] In the last SEER database, the reported incidence of thymic NETs was 0.02/100,000 population per year.[3] The median age at diagnosis is about 54 years with a male prevalence (male-to-female ratio of 3:1).[2,3]

Up to 25% of thymic NETs arise in patients with multiple endocrine neoplasia type 1 (MEN-1),[4,5] and among them, 3% to 8% develop thymic NETs.[5,6] Nearly all cases associated with MEN-1 are men and smokers.[7]

CLASSIFICATION

Despite the suggestion of benign behavior implied by their name, thymic carcinoids have been noted to present a more aggressive biologic behavior than their counterparts in other sites.

Wick and Rosai[8] suggested that the terms carcinoid and atypical carcinoid were outmoded and that such tumors should be regarded as part of the spectrum of neuroendocrine carcinomas.

Thymic carcinoids are rare tumors, which most closely resemble well-differentiated neuroendocrine carcinomas (atypical carcinoid tumors) of the lung in their histologic appearance and behavior. It has been argued by some that carcinoid tumors should also be classified as a type of thymic carcinoma (TC) for the following reasons[9]:

- They are not associated with paraneoplastic syndromes, which, conversely, frequently accompany thymoma
- They tend to metastasize to lymph nodes and extrathoracic organs, as do TCs
- The prognosis is similar to that of thymic carcinoma (one-third alive at 5 years)
- A carcinoid component occurs occasionally in other types of TCs

CLINICAL FEATURES

Clinical behavior closely correlated with the histologic degree of differentiation; disease-free survival was 50% at 5 years and 9% at 10 years for the well-differentiated tumors, 20% at 5 years, and 0% at 10 years for the moderately differentiated tumors, and 0% at 5 years for the poorly differentiated tumors.[10]

One-third of patients are asymptomatic, and the lesions may be discovered accidentally by imaging

[a] Department of Thoracic Surgery, University of Torino, Via Genova 3, Torino 10126, Italy; [b] Unit of Thoracic Surgery, Ospedali Riuniti, Via Conca 1, Ancona 60120, Italy; [c] Department of Thoracic Surgery, St James University Hospital, Beckett Street, Leeds LS9 7TF, UK
* Corresponding author.
E-mail address: alexit_2000@yahoo.com

Thorac Surg Clin 24 (2014) 327–332
http://dx.doi.org/10.1016/j.thorsurg.2014.05.007
1547-4127/14/$ – see front matter © 2014 Elsevier Inc. All rights reserved.

performed for other reasons or during MEN-1 surveillance.[2] Not infrequently, distant metastases are present at the time of diagnosis. Symptoms are due to the displacement or compression of thoracic organs, to associated endocrinopathies, or to the presence of distant metastases and may vary according to the extent of the disease, ranging from cough, dyspnea, chest pain, to superior vena cava syndrome (in approximately 20% of cases), and hoarseness from invasion of the recurrent laryngeal nerve. Thymic NETs are frequently associated with endocrinopathies and hormonal hypersecretions, such as adrenocorticotropic hormone (ACTH) ectopic production (Cushing syndrome, 10% of patients), growth hormone releasing hormone, hypersecretion with ectopic acromegaly, and hypertrophic osteoarthropathy.[11]

Other symptoms are sporadically reported: hyponatremia (due to the syndrome of inappropriate antidiuretic hormone [SIADH]) or atrial natriuretic peptide production. Other less commonly paraneoplastic conditions associated with these tumors are polyarthropathy, proximal myopathy, peripheral neuropathy, hypertrophic osteoarthropathy, and Lambert-Eaton syndrome. Myasthenia gravis (MG), which is the commonest paraneoplastic syndrome in thymoma, has been rarely described: an incidental thymic carcinoid tumor was observed in a man with a MG-associated thymoma.[12] The carcinoid syndrome has never been described.

Diagnostic workup includes chest radiographs, computed tomography (CT) scan, somatostatin receptor scintigraphy (**Fig. 1**), in selected cases, particularly in those with ectopic hormone production (eg, Cushing syndrome, SIADH). [18]Fluorodeoxy glucose positron emission tomography (PET) scan often shows false-negative results but might be positive in more aggressive and high-proliferation tumors as well as PET scanning with [68]Gallium-DOTATATE. Contrast-enhanced CT or magnetic resonance imaging (MRI) is recommended to detect possible tumor invasion in neighboring mediastinal tissues/organs (**Fig. 2**) as well as tumor metastases.

The diagnosis is made by histologic examination of tumor tissue supported by immunohistochemical neuroendocrine markers detection.

For thymic tumors diagnosis, mediastinotomy/thoracotomy may be sometimes required, even if recently transthoracic tru-cut biopsy (**Fig. 3**) was demonstrated to be effective.

The differential diagnosis includes other primary mediastinal tumors, mainly thymoma, paraganglioma, lymphoma, parathyroid adenoma or carcinoma, thymolipoma, soft tissue tumors, germ cell tumors, and medullary carcinoma of the thyroid arising in the mediastinal location.

The most difficult differential diagnosis in this setting is with thymoma, particularly the spindle cell type. The use of immunohistochemical stains can be helpful in such instances; thymomas will be negative for neuroendocrine markers such as chromogranin or synaptophysin. Mediastinal paragangliomas also may pose difficulties for diagnosis because of their prominent organoid or neuroendocrine growth pattern and positive staining for neuroendocrine markers. Immunohistochemical stains may be of aid in such instances; although both lesions share positivity for neuroendocrine markers such as synaptophysin and chromogranin, mediastinal paragangliomas are usually negative for CAM 5.2 cytokeratins.[13]

Carcinoid tumors metastatic to the thymus from another site are usually not occult, but search for

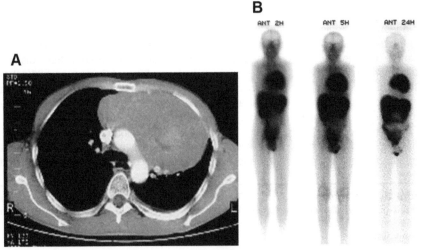

Fig. 1. Giant thymic neuroendocrine tumor: preoperative assessment. (*A*) Thoracic CT scan. (*B*) Octreotide scintigraphy.

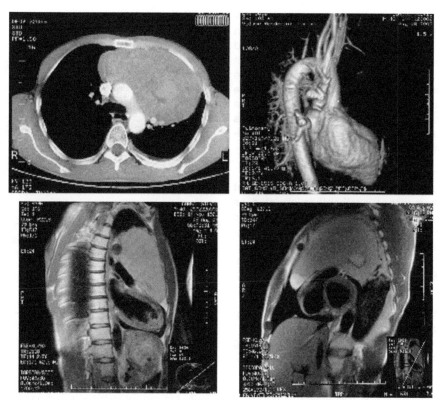

Fig. 2. Thymic neuroendocrine tumor: thoracic CT scan and MRI show the compression (but not the invasion) of the heart.

an extrathymic primary site should be done before diagnosing a thymic carcinoid tumor.

Other neuroendocrine neoplasms that may enter the differential diagnosis are ectopic mediastinal parathyroid tumors, including ectopic parathyroid adenomas and carcinomas. Immunohistochemical stains for parathyroid hormones also may be helpful for identifying these tumors in equivocal cases.

Medullary thyroid carcinoma arising in an ectopic mediastinal location also could be confused with a thymic neuroendocrine carcinoma. Positivity for calcitonin and carcinoembryonic antigen will help distinguish these lesions from primary mediastinal neuroendocrine carcinomas. Inclusion of lymphoid markers, such as leukocyte common antigen, L26, and UCHL-1, however, may be justified in the panel of immunostains used in cases showing the diffuse growth pattern to rule out the possibility of a lymphoid malignant neoplasm.

The biochemical profile for thymic carcinoid is usually similar to that of bronchial carcinoid.

Histologic Features

Rosai and Higa[14] were the first to acknowledge the existence of carcinoid tumors in the thymus and to separate them from more common tumors arising in this site, such as thymoma.

They also pointed out that previous reports[15,16] on thymomas associated with endocrine abnormalities most likely corresponded to cases of primary neuroendocrine tumors of the thymus.

Another interesting finding observed in the high-grade lesions was the presence of areas showing

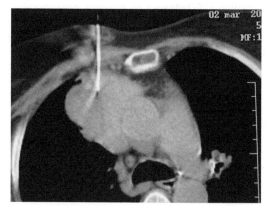

Fig. 3. Transthoracic CT-guided biopsy of an invasive thymic carcinoid.

features of well-differentiated neuroendocrine carcinoma of the thymus (classic thymic carcinoid) in direct transition with areas of poorly differentiated neuroendocrine carcinoma indistinguishable from those of small cell (oat cell) carcinoma of the lung.[17] The existence of such cases supports the notion that these tumors represent part of a continuous spectrum of differentiation that ranges from typical, well-differentiated carcinoid to small-cell neuroendocrine carcinoma type 2.[10]

Gross features

Tumors usually do not have a capsule and the cut surface is homogeneous rather than lobulated, as is characteristic of thymomas. The cut surfaces are usually firm and gray; focal necrosis and hemorrhage are also frequent (**Fig. 4**).[18]

The World Health Organization classification of thymic NETs classifies these tumors into 2 groups[19]:

1. Well-differentiated thymic NETs (including typical and atypical carcinoids)
2. Poorly differentiated thymic NETs (including large cell neuroendocrine carcinoma [LCNC] and small cell carcinoma [SCC]).

Under the microscope, well-differentiated NETs present monotonous cells with abundant cytoplasm, small round nuclei, and modest nucleoli. Atypical carcinoids present with more frequent areas of necrosis and higher proliferative rate. On the other hand, poorly differentiated NETs are characterized by large (LCNC) or small (SCC) cells with cytologic atypias and nucleal chromatin that may lead to the artifact of nucleal material.

Several variants include a usual form and diffuse, spindled, desmoplastic (fibrotic), and mucinous types, as well as a variant resembling medullary carcinoma of the thyroid.[18] A proliferation of pigmented thymic melanocytes darkened the gross appearance of one tumor.[20]

Immunohistochemistry

The tumors often show architectural features of neuroendocrine differentiation. Tumors react with antibodies to cytokeratin and chromogranin A, as well as other neuroendocrine markers, including synaptophysin, CD56, and Leu-7. In addition, tumors may show reactivity for ACTH, serotonin, calcitonin, gastrin, cholecystokinin, or somatostatin, even if there is no clinical evidence of their presence.

Electron microscopy

Similar to bronchial carcinoids, thymic carcinoid tumors have neurosecretory granules. These tumors range in size from 100 to 400 nm.[18]

TREATMENT AND OUTCOME
Management of Localized Disease

Thymic NETs should be referred to an experienced center for careful evaluation and treatment. A particular approach in a multidisciplinary setting is also advisable.

Thymic NETs should whenever feasible be subjected to radical surgical resection. Unfortunately, the percentage of recurrence remained remarkably high, higher than in bronchial NET counterparts, and a life-long follow-up is recommended also in radically operated patients.

The prognosis remains poor due to the aggressive nature of the tumor with a high incidence of recurrence following surgery. Low-grade thymic NETs present 5-year and 10-year survival rates of 50% and 9%, respectively, whereas no high grade survives at 5 years.[11]

Management of Advanced/Metastatic Disease

An aggressive multidisciplinary treatment (usually induction CT, followed by surgery, postoperative CT, and/or radiotherapy) is indicated in the case of an advanced lesion.[18,19] Resection of the primary tumor along with invaded mediastinal organs/tissues is generally performed. Median sternotomy is the commonest intervention, although sometimes combined access (sternotomy + anterior thoracotomy) or thoracotomy is indicated according to the scheduled type of resection.

Cytotoxic treatment combined with surgical resection when indicated has been the standard for metastatic thymic NETs, although the available chemotherapy regimens demonstrate a rather poor effect.[21,22]

Response to chemotherapy or radiation alone is poor. Embolic metastases occur in up to

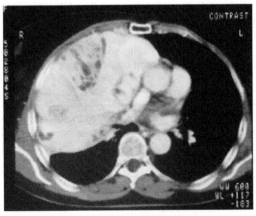

Fig. 4. Giant right-sided neuroendocrine tumor of the thymus: hemorrhagic/necrotic areas within the lesion are evident.

three-fourths of patients. Metastatic sites include mediastinal lymph nodes, but distant metastases (bone, liver, skin) occur in 30% to 40% of cases.[8]

Symptomatic metastatic disease confined to the liver may be treated with embolization, radiofrequency ablation, and radioembolization. External brain and bone metastases irradiation might also be beneficial.

Classic cisplatinum-based chemotherapy regimen is reported to be effective, although temozolomide is a new promising drug, currently used in advanced neuroendocrine tumors.[23,24]

In low-proliferating and functional tumors, the treatment with somatostatin analogues[25] and α-interferons might also be an option. In nonfunctional ones, their use is still controversial.

Differences in 5-year survival have been observed between thymic NETs without and with endocrinopathies (70% vs 35%, respectively).[8]

There is a lack of standard treatment for thymic malignancies after failure of platinum-based chemotherapy and, in this scenario, alternative therapeutic molecular targets are being developed. Recent molecular characterization of thymoma and TC includes identification of several oncogenes (EGFR, HER2, KIT, KRAS, and BCL2), tumor suppressor genes (TP53, p16INK4A), chromosomal aberrations (LOH 3p, 6p, 6q, 7p, 8p), angiogenetic factors (vascular endothelial growth factor), and tumor invasion factors (matrix metalloproteinases and tissue inhibitors of metalloproteinases) involved in tumor growth and proliferation. Based on the efficacy previously shown in many other solid tumors, several molecular targeted therapies have been evaluated in phase II clinical trials.

In particular, different tyrosine kinase inhibitors, angiogenesis inhibitors, histone deacetylase inhibitors, DNA methyltransferase inhibitors, and cyclin-dependent kinases/tropomyosin receptor kinase A inhibitors have shown some activity in thymomas and in TC.

Because of the lack of data, adequate-sized prospective trials are required for validation, and the enrollment of patients with advanced disease into available clinical trials must be encouraged.[26]

REFERENCES

1. Goto K, Kodama T, Matsuno Y, et al. Clinicopathologic and DNA cytometric analysis of carcinoid tumors of the thymus. Mod Pathol 2001;14:985–94.
2. Chaer R, Massad MG, Evans A, et al. Primary neuroendocrine tumors of the thymus. Ann Thorac Surg 2002;74:1733–40.
3. Gaur P, Leary C, Yao JC. Thymic neuroendocrine tumors: a SEER database analysis of 160 patients. Ann Surg 2010;251:1117–21.
4. Teh BT, McArdle J, Chan SP, et al. Clinicopathologic studies of thymic carcinoids in multiple endocrine neoplasia type 1. Medicine (Baltimore) 1997;76:21–9.
5. Gibril F, Chen YJ, Schrump DS, et al. Prospective study of thymic carcinoids in patients with multiple endocrine neoplasia type 1. J Clin Endocrinol Metab 2003;88:1066–81.
6. Ferolla P, Falchetti A, Filosso P, et al. Thymic neuroendocrine carcinoma (carcinoid) in multiple endocrine neoplasia type 1 syndrome: the Italian series. J Clin Endocrinol Metab 2005;90:2603–9.
7. Goudet P, Bonithon-Kopp C, Murat A, et al. Gender-related differences in MEN1 lesion occurrence and diagnosis: a cohort study of 734 cases from the Groupe d'etude des Tumeurs Endocrines. Eur J Endocrinol 2011;165(1):97–105.
8. Wick MR, Rosai J. Neuroendocrine neoplasms of the thymus. Pathol Res Pract 1988;183:188–99.
9. de Montpréville V, Macchiarini P, Dulmet E. Thymic neuroendocrine carcinoma (carcinoid): a clinicopathologic study of fourteen cases. J Thorac Cardiovasc Surg 1996;111:134–41.
10. Moran CA, Suster S. Neuroendocrine carcinomas (carcinoid tumor) of the thymus: a clinicopathologic analysis of 80 cases. Am J Clin Pathol 2000;114:100–10.
11. Phan AT, Oberg K, Choi J, et al. NANETS consensus guideline for the diagnosis and management of neuroendocrine tumors: well-differentiated neuroendocrine tumors of the thorax (includes lung and thymus). Pancreas 2010;39(6):784–98.
12. Mizuno T, Masaoka A, Hashimoto T, et al. Coexisting thymic carcinoid tumor and thymoma. Ann Thorac Surg 1990;50:650–2.
13. Moran CA, Suster S, Fishback N, et al. Mediastinal paragangliomas: a clinicopathologic and immunohistochemical study of 16 cases. Cancer 1993;72:2358–64.
14. Rosai J, Higa E. Mediastinal endocrine neoplasm of probable thymic origin related to carcinoid tumor. Cancer 1972;29:1061–74.
15. Kay S, Willson MA. Ultrastructural studies of an ACTH secreting thymic tumor. Cancer 1970;26:445–52.
16. Duguid JB, Kennedy AM. Oat-cell tumours of mediastinal glands. J Pathol 1930;23:93–9.
17. Wick MR, Scheithauer BW. Oat-cell carcinoma of the thymus. Cancer 1982;49:1652–7.
18. Wick M, Rosai J. Neuroendocrine neoplasms of the mediastinum. Semin Diagn Pathol 1991;8:35–51.
19. Marx A, Shimosato Y, Kuo TT, et al. Thymic neuroendocrine tumours. In: Travis WD, Brambilla E, Muller-Hermelink HK, et al, editors. Pathology & genetics: tumours of the lung, pleura, thymus and heart. Lyon (France): IARC Press; 2004. p. 188–95.

20. Ho F, Ho J. Pigmented carcinoid tumour of the thymus. Histopathology 1977;1:363–9.

21. Oberg K. Chemotherapy and biotherapy in the treatment of neuroendocrine tumors. Ann Oncol 2001;12: S111–4.

22. Hamada S, Masago K, Mio T, et al. Good clinical response to imatinib mesylate in atypical thymic carcinoid with KIT overexpression. J Clin Oncol 2011;29:e9–10.

23. Ekeblad S, Sundin A, Janson ET, et al. Temozolomide as monotherapy is effective in treatment of advanced malignant neuroendocrine tumors. Clin Cancer Res 2007;13:2986–91.

24. van Essen M, Krenning EP, Bakker WH, et al. Peptide receptor radionuclide therapy with 177Lu-octreotate in patients with foregut carcinoid tumors of bronchial, gastric and thymic origin. Eur J Nucl Med Mol Imaging 2007;34(8):1219–27.

25. Filosso PL, Actis Dato GM, Ruffini E, et al. Multidisciplinary treatment of advanced thymic neuroendocrine carcinoma (carcinoid): report of a successful case and review of the literature. J Thorac Cardiovasc Surg 2004;127:1215–9.

26. Kondo K, Monden Y. Therapy for thymic epithelial tumors: a clinical study of 1320 patients from Japan. Ann Thorac Surg 2003;76:878–84.

Peptide Receptor Radionuclide Therapy for Advanced Neuroendocrine Tumors

Lisa Bodei, MD, PhD[a],*, Marta Cremonesi, PhD[b], Mark Kidd, PhD[c],
Chiara M. Grana, MD[a], Stefano Severi, MD[d],
Irvin M. Modlin, MD, PhD, DSc, MA, FRCS (Eng. & Ed), FCS (SA)[c,e],
Giovanni Paganelli, MD[a,d]

KEYWORDS

- Bone marrow • Bronchopulmonary • Carcinoid • Gastroenteropancreatic neuroendocrine tumor
- Hepatic neuroendocrine metastasis • Peptide receptor radionuclide therapy • PRRT • Renal toxicity

KEY POINTS

- Peptide receptor radionuclide therapy (PRRT) with either ^{90}Y-octreotide or ^{177}Lu-octreotate is an efficient and relatively safe treatment of unresectable or metastatic neuroendocrine tumors.
- Over 2 decades, PRRT has been demonstrated to provide effective tumor response, symptom relief, and quality-of-life improvement, biomarker reduction, and, ultimately, a positive impact on survival.
- PRRT is generally well tolerated. Chronic and permanent effects on target organs, particularly the kidneys and the bone marrow, are generally mild if appropriate precautions are undertaken.

INTRODUCTION

Neuroendocrine neoplasms are variously referred to as "carcinoids," neuroendocrine tumors (NETs), or gastroenteropancreatic (GEP) neuroendocrine (NE) neoplasms (GEP-NENs).[1] Most NETs are located in the gastroenteropancreatic tract and in the lung (**Fig. 1**).[1] In general, they are slow-growing tumors but in some instances may behave in a highly aggressive fashion (neuroendocrine carcinoma; NEC).[2] Due to their diverse and protean symptoms (sweating, flushing, diarrhea, bronchospasm, and anxiety), diagnosis is often significantly delayed and lesions therefore are only identified when metastatic spread has occurred. Metastasis can occur locally, in the mesentery, in adjacent lymph nodes, and by hematogenous spread. In most, the liver is the dominant site of metastatic spread, but lung, bone, and brain may also be affected.[3] As a consequence of the substantial percentage of individuals with metastatic disease, most therapeutic strategies are directed at the management of hepatic secondaries or local recurrence.[4]

Given the different organ distribution of the primaries and their widely different biologic behavior, treatment of NETs is typically multidisciplinary and is individualized according to the tumor type,

The authors have nothing to disclose.
[a] Division of Nuclear Medicine, European Institute of Oncology, via Ripamonti 435, Milan 20141, Italy;
[b] Division of Health Physics, European Institute of Oncology, via Ripamonti 435, Milan 20141, Italy;
[c] Department of Surgery, Yale School of Medicine, 310 Cedar Street, New Haven, CT 06520, USA;
[d] Radiometabolic Unit, Department of Nuclear Medicine, IRST-IRCCS, Via Maroncelli 40, Meldola 47014, Italy; [e] Clifton Life Sciences, Branford, CT 06405, USA
* Corresponding author.
E-mail address: lisa.bodei@ieo.it

Thorac Surg Clin 24 (2014) 333–349
http://dx.doi.org/10.1016/j.thorsurg.2014.04.005

thoracic.theclinics.com

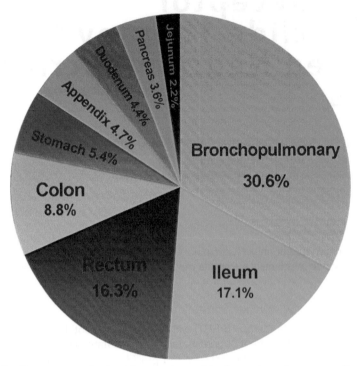

Fig. 1. Incidence of different types of NETs. Most are located in the gastroenteropancreatic tract and the lung.

extent of the disease, and level of symptoms. GEP-NENs were previously considered rare, but in fact, not only are increasing in incidence (3.65/100,000), but also occur as frequently as testicular tumors, Hodgkin disease, gliomas, and multiple myeloma.[1] They represent a significant clinical issue for 2 reasons. First, at diagnosis, 40% to 95% are metastatic (depending on the primary site) and, second, there is a paucity of evidence-based best practice strategies.[1] A key management issue is that at diagnosis, 65% to 95% of GEP-NENs (excluding appendiceal and gastric NETs) have metastasized to the liver.[5,6] Therapeutic endeavors are therefore in most instances focused on the management of metastatic disease, and neuroendocrine liver metastases (NE LMs) represent one of the most significant prognostic factors irrespective of the primary tumor site. Thus, the 5-year survival in historical series is 13% to 54% compared with 75% to 99% in individuals without hepatic metastases.[7,8]

Recent experience from some specialized centers documents improved 5-year overall survival rates of 56% to 83% for metastasized intestinal NENs and 40% to 60% for pancreatic NENs.[9] Although these data have been used to suggest that NET management should only be undertaken at specialized centers, such proposals may not be realistic in the current medical economic climate. Despite the use of a diverse variety of complex management strategies for NE LMs, surgery

remains the only treatment option with the potential to cure.[9] For unresectable tumors, optimal selection of palliative treatment options (timing and modality) is of paramount importance to maintain or improve quality of life (QoL) and prolong overall survival.

OVERVIEW

Unlike many well-studied neoplastic diseases such as breast or colon cancer, NETs represent relatively recent clinicopathologic entities. As a consequence, their management has evolved over the last decade based on increased understanding of their tumor biology and molecular regulation. Given the diverse appreciation of the disease complexity, a variety of different sequences of diagnostic and therapeutic procedures has being proposed and debated in individual medical centers.[10] Key issues involved in the development of an optimal management strategy include the precise type of the tumor, the grade and stage of the lesion, and the overall patient's general condition. Ideally, removal of the primary tumor should be initially undertaken and, thereafter, appropriate strategies should be developed for the management of residual disease. It is the latter issue that often evokes controversial discussion because there exists a paucity of rigorous prospective randomized trials to support a clearly defined therapeutic strategy. In most cases, therefore, the therapeutic strategy is usually determined by discussion based on experience and institutional bias.[10] Although a variety of management guidelines have been developed, they tend to vary from country to country. The most significant limitation of the published recommendations is that, in most circumstances, they are based on low-grade evidence obtained from retrospective studies of heterogeneous patient and tumor populations.[4]

In principle, however, the choice of therapy depends on the primary therapeutic aim for a particular individual, which may range from an attempt at complete surgical eradication of the disease to amelioration of symptoms. In most circumstances, complete removal of disease is impossible because of a late clinical presentation with evidence of metastatic progression (**Fig. 2**). The latter may be local or more commonly involves hepatic metastasis and occasionally spread to bone, lungs, and even brain. Thus, for practical clinical purposes, most therapy is deployed toward decreasing the size of metastatic lesions, reducing metastatic growth, and ameliorating symptoms (in functional lesions).[11] To achieve these goals, a wide variety of therapeutic strategies have been developed. The surgical options include resection

of the primary, hepatic metastases resection, radiofrequency ablation, and even hepatic transplantation.[12] Interventional radiology techniques include embolization of hepatic metastases (with or without cytotoxic agents) or the use of radioactive microspheres. Medical therapy ranges from the use of bioactive agents such as somatostatin analogues or interferon to standard chemotherapy. More recently, a variety of novel molecular targeted agents, including Everolimus, Sunitinib, and Bevacuzimab, have been used with marginal efficacy.[13] Of particular interest has been the development of targeted radiotherapy using a variety of different isotopes, including indium, yttrium, and lutetium.[14] This novel therapeutic strategy, delivered by intravenous infusion, has been designated peptide receptor radionuclide therapy (PRRT) (**Fig. 3**).

NON-SOMATOSTATIN-BASED THERAPIES
Medical Therapy

In general, the type of therapy used depends on the grade and proliferation of the tumor. High-grade, rapidly proliferating lesions, especially from the pancreas (NEC G3), are amenable to chemotherapy, whereas "targeted" therapies (eg,

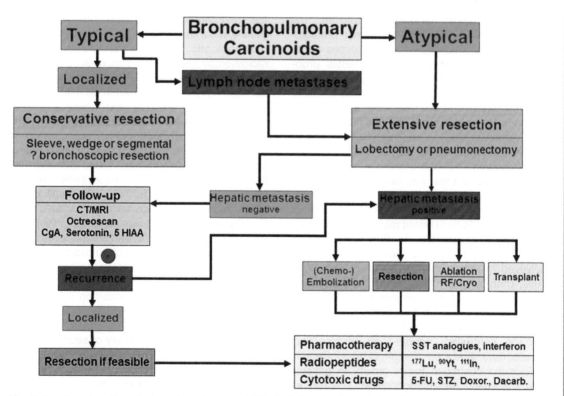

Fig. 2. Treatment options in bronchopulmonary NETs, including both typical and atypical carcinoids. The management of metastatic or unresectable disease comprises locoregional strategies as well as systemic treatments, including PRRT.

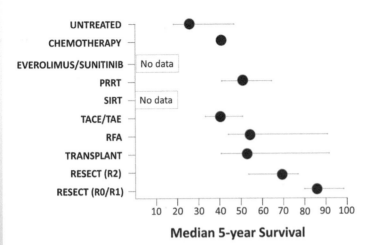

Fig. 3. Treatment outcomes for NETs. Therapy-related survival is the highest in resectable tumors. At diagnosis, 40% to 95% of tumors have already metastasized (depending on location of the primary lesion). PRRT compares well with other techniques, including locoregional approaches and chemotherapy. Toxicity is a major adverse event in the latter category of therapy.

Everolimus or Sunitinib) and biotherapy (eg, somatostatin analogues or interferon) are used in "slower" growing lesions (NET G1 or G2). Chemotherapy has greater objective response rates (35%–40%) in pancreatic NETs than Everolimus or Sunitinib.[15] The molecular markers that identify patients who would optimally benefit from individual or combinations of therapies, apart from somatostatin receptor expression, are currently unknown. For chemotherapy (including 5-fluorouracil, doxorubicin, and streptozotocin), the volume of LM is the most significant predictor of outcome and directly correlates with progression-free survival (PFS). Potential problems with chemotherapy include cumulative risks of nephrotoxicity/myelosuppression and systemic adverse events.[16] For targeted therapies, there is evidence to suggest a specific use in NE LMs. In the Everolimus study in pancreatic NETs, 92% of whom had NE LMs, the agent was associated with improved PFS (6.4 months compared with placebo), an effect that was long lasting (35% stable at 18 months). Tumor remissions were, however, rare (5%). In the Sunitinib study (95% of pancreatic NETs had distant metastases including NE LMs), a significant PFS prolongation (5.9 months compared with placebo) was achieved with tumor remissions of less than 10%. There is no evidence for use of Sunitinib or Everolimus in LM of intestinal origin. For biotherapies, there is a modest amount of data for interferon, but for somatostatin analogues, the Placebo controlled, double-blind, prospective, Randomized study on the effect of Octreotide LAR in the control of tumor growth in patients with metastatic neuroendocrine MIDgut tumors (PROMID) study on small bowel NETs suggested that any benefit from these agents was defined by the extent of liver involvement. Thus, individuals with less than 10% involvement had better PFS than those with greater than 10% involvement. In summary, 3 prospective randomized trials provide only marginal evidence for the efficacy of these agents (Everolimus and Sunitinib) in the treatment of NE LMs.

Angiographic Liver-directed Techniques

Liver-directed intra-arterial therapies available in the treatment of unresectable NE LMs include trans-arterial embolization (TAE), transarterial chemoembolization (TACE), and selective internal radiotherapy (SIRT) with Yttrium-90 (^{90}Y) microspheres. For TAE or TACE, symptomatic responses have been reported in 53% to 100% of patients (10–55 months) and morphologic responses were noted in 35% to 74% (6–63 months) with a PFS of ~18 months with 5-year survivals of 40% to 83%. Mortality and morbidity, including postembolization syndrome, varied between 0% to 5.6% and 28% to 90%, respectively; TAE appears to be superior to TACE for small bowel NETs. In a recent multicenter report on SIRT, stable disease by imaging was achieved in 22.7%, a partial response in 60.5%, and complete response in 2.7%. A median survival of 70 months was reported with progressive disease evident in 4.9%. The most frequently observed clinical toxicities were fatigue and nausea (occurring in <10%). In an international multicenter prospective treatment registry to investigate the safety and efficacy of hepatic artery therapy for primary or secondary liver tumors, response rates for SIRT and TACE were comparable at 6 months in a group of 43 patients with comparable NE LM disease. At 12 months, however, a significantly lower response rate was observed in the SIRT group: 46% versus 66%. Although SIRT may have advantages over TAE/

TACE in terms of reduced adverse effects and the requirement for fewer treatments, it can be associated with side effects in terms of radiation gastritis, duodenal ulceration, and sclerotic alteration of healthy liver parenchyma. SIRT is also relatively expensive and patients require careful selection because lung shunting may be an issue. It is clear that more long-term outcome data are required to assess the efficacy of SIRT.

SOMATOSTATIN ANALOGUE-RELATED THERAPIES

"Cold," non-radiolabeled, somatostatin analogues exhibit significant effects in terms of ameliorating symptoms. The various synthetic peptide analogues each have different binding properties to the 5 somatostatin receptor subtypes. Generally, however, they represent an effective class of agents that inhibit peptide secretion from NET cells with relatively few and limited adverse events.[17] This is particularly evident in small bowel NETs, which often exhibit severe flushing and diarrhea. Similar positive effects are evident in functional pancreatic NETs, such as glucagonoma and VIPoma. Unfortunately, administration requires monthly injections, which are inconvenient and often painful. Furthermore, the beneficial pharmacologic effects are not always sustained (breakthrough) because of either tachyphylaxis or increasing production of bioactive products by an advancing tumor.[18] It has been proposed that cold somatostatin analogues decrease proliferative activity of NETs. The evidence for this

assertion is, however, neither rigorous nor robust and, if such an effect is present, it is only evident in a small minority of lesions.[19,20]

PRRT with radiolabeled somatostatin analogues is an innovative treatment of inoperable or metastasized, well/moderately differentiated, NETs, particularly of the GEP (and of the lung).[21] Somatostatin analogues represent, to date, the prototype and the most successful paradigm of radiopeptide therapy. This successful paradigm of radiopeptide therapy reflects the development of a synthetic peptide analogue, octreotide, and its variants, using the native somatostatin molecule as a base. Overall, the therapeutic efficacy of somatostatin analogues and, subsequently, of their radiolabeled counterparts, is due to their high affinity for somatostatin receptors subtype 2 (S2) and moderate affinity for subtype 5 (S5) and is consistent with the prevalent overexpression of S2 and S5 in most NETs.[22]

PRRT Background

The rational scientific PRRT basis relies in the presence of a somatostatin receptor on the surface of NETs to which an isotopically labeled radiopeptide is directed. The subsequent cellular radiopeptide internalization thereafter delivers the radioactivity directly into the intracellular compartment of the tumor (**Fig. 4**). The clinical process of PRRT consists in the systemic administration of a suitably radiolabeled synthetic somatostatin analogue, fractionated in sequential cycles (usually 4–5) every 6 to 9 weeks, until

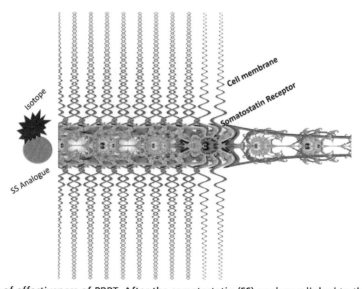

Fig. 4. Mechanism of effectiveness of PRRT. After the somatostatin (SS) analogue linked to the isotope binds to the membrane somatostatin receptor, the radiopeptide/somatostatin receptor complex is internalized. Thus, radioactivity is transported into the intracellular receptor recycling compartment of the NET cell, where it exerts its action in proximity to the nucleus.

the intended total amount of radioactivity has been delivered. The precise amount administered depends mainly on the limitations imposed by renal irradiation and to a lesser extent on bone marrow.

PRRT was introduced into clinical practice in 1994. It represented a logical step following the initial development of the diagnostic technique for in vivo localization of NETs using the radiolabeled somatostatin analogue [^{111}In-DTPA0-D-Phe1]-octreotide or ^{111}In-pentetreotide.[23] Thus, the same principle was used, but increased isotope activity (high-dose ^{111}In-pentetreotide) provided a therapeutic as opposed to a diagnostic benefit. Therapeutic efficacy reflects the activity of the Auger and conversion electrons emitted by ^{111}In. Despite the theoretical considerations, partial remissions remained rare.[24] As a consequence of these relatively disappointing results, isotopes with higher energy and longer range, such as the pure β emitter ^{90}Y, were considered more appropriate for therapeutic evaluation. The β particles emitted by ^{90}Y (maximum energy 2.27 MeV, penetration range $R_{\beta max}$ 11 mm, half-life $T_{1/2}$ 64 hours) are advantageous, allowing simultaneously a direct killing of somatostatin receptor-positive cells and a cross-fire effect that targets nearby receptor-negative tumor cells. To facilitate efficacy further, novel octreotide analogues were developed. Thus, for ^{90}Y, a new analogue, Tyr^3-octreotide, with a similar pattern of affinity for somatostatin receptors, was developed at the University of Basel. This analogue was characterized by high hydrophobicity, ease of labeling with ^{111}In and ^{90}Y, and tight binding to the bifunctional chelator DOTA, which securely encloses the radioisotope (1,4,7,10-tetra-azacyclododecane-N,N',N'',N'''-tetra-acetic acid).[25,26]

[^{90}Y-DOTA^0,Tyr^3]-octreotide or ^{90}Y-DOTATOC or ^{90}Y-octreotide was initially used in the treatment of metastatic NETs in 1996. The excellent symptomatic and objective response following several cycles of ^{90}Y-octreotide therapy encouraged further studies to examine the potential of PRRT in NET disease.[27] As a consequence of the positive experience with ^{90}Y-octreotide, it became the most used radiopeptide in the first decade of PRRT experience.[14,28–31]

Since 2000, however, a more effective analogue, octreotate (Tyr^3, Thr^8-octreotide), with 6-fold to 9-fold higher affinity for somatostatin S2 has been used. The chelated analogue [DOTA]^0-Tyr^3-octreotate or DOTATATE can be labeled with the β-γ emitter Lutetium-177 (E$_{\beta max}$ 0.49 MeV, $R_{\beta max}$ 2 mm, $T_{1/2}$ 6.7 days) and has been investigated in several clinical phase I and II studies **(Fig. 5)**.[14,32–34] ^{177}Lu-octreotate has

subsequently become one of the most frequently used radiopeptides for PRRT; this has been particularly evident in recent years given its efficacy, tolerability, and manageability. ^{177}Lu-octreotate is currently being evaluated in a randomized phase III registration trial in small bowel NETs.

PRRT Clinical Protocol

Candidates for PRRT with radiolabeled somatostatin analogues are individuals with tumors that exhibit a significant somatostatin receptor overexpression. A key issue in the inclusion criteria is that the somatostatin receptors should be functional, namely, be able to internalize the receptor-analogue complex and retain the radioactivity inside the cell. Thus, the critical issues for effective therapy remain the somatostatin receptor overexpression and the evidence of functionality.

To be considered appropriate candidates for therapy, individuals should be selected based on scintigraphy with ^{111}In-pentetreotide (or, more recently, receptor positron emission tomography [PET] with ^{68}Gallium-labeled octreotide). Such images should indicate an adequate uptake (at least equal to the uptake of normal liver) as evidence of adequate expression of targetable somatostatin receptors; this is necessary to ensure and calculate an appropriate high tumor dose with low

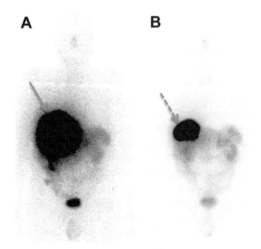

A   **B**

Fig. 5. Objective response to ^{177}Lu-octreotate PRRT in an unresectable rectal NET with hepatic metastasis (*A*) basal ^{177}Lu-octreotate scan (*solid arrow*). The patient underwent a prior rectosigmoid resection and exhibited disease progression following chemotherapy with capecitabine. (*B*) The final ^{177}Lu-octreotate scan after 8.6 GBq of ^{177}Lu-octreotate. Evidence of a partial objective response (*dashed arrow*) enabled subsequent embolization followed by a multidisciplinary treatment sequence plan.

exposure to normal tissues that express physiologic levels of somatostatin receptors.[35]

Scintigraphic or PET tomoscintigraphic evaluation is to date the most accurate noninvasive method to identify and confirm the overexpression of functioning receptors. An alternative strategy is to use immunohistochemistry, which provides similar information at the time of biopsy. Immunohistochemistry, however, is not as quantitatively accurate as molecular analysis (polymerase chain reaction and Western blot), which can precisely define the level of somatostatin receptors and their functionality.[36] Optimally, the use of in vivo functional scintigraphic or PET methods facilitates the simultaneous evaluation of the receptor density and the internalization capacity in real-time in all lesions.

When evaluating a receptor scan to determine PRRT selection, it is important to exclude false positives. For the most part, these represent accumulations of inflammatory cells, which express somatostatin receptors. False positives include gallbladder (inflammation), accessory spleens, recent surgical scars (inflammatory infiltrate), previous radiotherapy, and any other cause of granulomatous-lymphoid infiltrate that can mimic the presence of NET tissue.

Potential causes of false negatives should also be considered. These false negatives are mainly represented by small, subcentimeter lesions, under the resolution limit of the instrument (although this limitation is partially overcome by receptor PET/computed tomography). In addition, certain tumors, especially benign insulinomas and most highly malignant NETs, do not express adequate somatostatin receptors for detection.

PRRT Technique

PRRT consists of the cyclical systemic administration of the radiopeptide. The cumulative activity, fractionated in multiple cycles, is able to irradiate the tumor efficiently, without surpassing the conventional 25- to 27-Gy absorbed dose threshold to the kidneys, which are the dose-limiting organs. Recently, it has been reported that the biologic effective dose (BED) as opposed to the absorbed dose provides a dose threshold value that is slightly higher.[37] The rhythm of fractionation, every 6 to 9 weeks, is based on the time that has been determined as necessary to recover from possible hematological toxicity.

To diminish the renal dose of irradiation, patients are premedicated with an intravenous infusion of positively charged amino acids (lysine or arginine) in the amount of at least 25 g per day. This infusion is started 2 to 3 hours before the isotope administration and is maintained until 2 to 3 hours following cessation of the isotope infusion. The infusion has the objective of simultaneously hydrating the patients and reducing the renal radioactivity dose by providing competitive inhibition of the proximal tubular reabsorption of the radiopeptide. The radiopeptide is intravenously administered slowly over 20 minutes in approximately 100 mL of saline. In some circumstances, mild adverse events are experienced during the infusion. These mild adverse events include gastrointestinal symptoms, such as a slight nausea, and occasionally, emesis. These symptoms may be related to the amino acid coadministration, but are easily controlled with appropriate medication.[21]

PRRT Efficacy

In almost 2 decades of clinical application, PRRT with ^{90}Y-octreotide or ^{177}Lu-octreotate has provided effective clinical therapy as indicated by tumor responses, symptom relief, and QoL improvement as well as a decrease in biomarker levels and enhanced survival (see **Fig. 5**). Several clinical phase I–II trials indicate that radiolabeled somatostatin analogue PRRT is among the promising newly developed targeted tools in NETs, with registered objective responses in more than 30% of individuals, mainly of GEP origin.[14,31,33,35,38–40]

PRRT and Bronchopulmonary NETs

Although bronchial NETs overall represent the second most common type of NET among differentiated histologic types, there have been few, dedicated PRRT trials. The PRRT data for bronchopulmonary NETs are therefore typically extrapolated from more general studies (**Fig. 6**).

In the first decade of experience, ^{90}Y-octreotide was the most commonly used radiopeptide. However, all the published results derive from different phase I–II studies performed independently by a variety of centers. As a consequence, information is heterogeneous as to inclusion criteria and specific treatment schemes. A rigorous direct comparison is therefore virtually impossible at this time. Nevertheless, despite these limitations, objective responses have been documented in 10% to 34% of patients (**Table 1**).[14,29,30,39–42]

Current isotope administration protocols schedule the injection of standard radioactivities that were established based on previous dose escalation studies as well as clinical experience. This practice has resulted in substantial differences among protocols, as to activities, which may be fixed or related to body weight or surface, number of cycles, and time intervals between cycles.

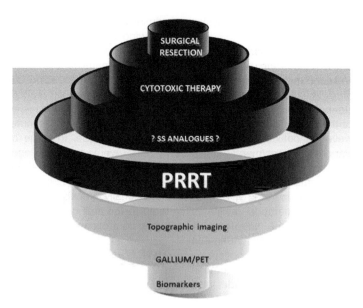

SURGICAL RESECTION

CYTOTOXIC THERAPY

? SS ANALOGUES ?

PRRT

Topographic imaging

GALLIUM/PET

Biomarkers

Fig. 6. Role of diagnostic and therapeutic tools in the management of bronchopulmonary NETs ranging from surgical resection to PRRT.

The initial studies with ^{90}Y-octreotide were undertaken in individuals with very advanced disease. However, the documented effectiveness of the therapy, even in these situations, led to the usage of PRRT in earlier phases of disease because it was evident that with decreased tumor burden radiopeptides exhibited a greater efficacy. The rationale for this strategy was provided by numerous factors including tumor volume and the biologic features of the neoplasm. Thus, more advanced (aggressive) tumors expressed less somatostatin receptors, increased genetic mutations, such as in p53,[43] and are thus less responsive to treatment. Key issues in predicting optimal PRRT outcome were tumor load,

especially in the liver, and performance status. Evaluation of such indices of prognosis and outcome concluded that treatment in a phase of "early" progression rather than a "wait-and-see" approach was advantageous. Overall, it was apparent that PRRT treatment in advanced stage disease was substantially less effective. A further consideration was the type of disease being treated. Thus, metastases of pancreatic NETs were frequently more amenable to therapy compared with other types of NETs. NETs that were active secretors of bioactive agents (functional) also tended to relapse very rapidly.[44]

In a study carried out at Basel University, 39 patients with NETs, mostly of GEP origin, were

Table 1
Clinical results of PRRT with either ^{90}Y-octreotide or ^{177}Lu-octreotate in GEP-NETs

Ligand (Ref.)	Patient Number	CR + PR (%)	Response Criteria	Outcome (mo)
[90]Y-octreotide[41]	23	13	WHO	Not assessed
[90]Y-octreotide[57]	37	27	WHO	TTP >26
[90]Y-octreotide[45]	36	34	WHO	Not assessed
[90]Y-octreotide[28]	21	29	WHO	TTP 10
[90]Y-octreotide[42]	58	9	SWOG	TTP 29
[90]Y-octreotide[30]	90	4	SWOG	PFS 16
[90]Y-octreotide[40]	53	23	WHO	PFS 29
[90]Y-octreotate[39]	58	23	WHO	PFS 17
[177]Lu-octreotate[33]	310	29	SWOG	PFS 33
[177]Lu-octreotate[34]	42	31	RECIST	TTP 36
[177]Lu-octreotate[52]	52	39	SWOG	PFS 29

treated with 4 cycles of ^{90}Y-octreotide, with a cumulative activity of 7.4 GBq. Objective responses, according to World Health Organization (WHO) criteria, were described in 23%, with a complete remission in 2 patients, a partial response in 7 patients, and a disease stabilization in 27 patients. Pancreatic NETs (13 patients) showed a better objective response (38% partial + complete) than other tumor types. A significant related-symptoms amelioration occurred in most patients. In this series, 3 patients with progressive bronchial tumors were also included. All demonstrated disease stabilization after PRRT.[45]

In a multicenter phase I study, carried out in Rotterdam, Louvain, and Tampa, 60 patients with GEP-NETs were treated with 4 cycles of 0.9, 1.8, 2.8, 3.7, 4.6, and 5.5 GBq/m^2 of ^{90}Y-octreotide administered at 6 to 9 weekly intervals. In an initial evaluation of the results (2002) in 32 evaluable patients, objective responses (according to Southwest Oncology Group [SWOG] criteria) were evident. These responses constituted ~9% partial responses and 9% minor responses.[46] In a subsequent reanalysis of 58 assessable patients of the same population who were treated with cumulative activities of 1.7 to 32.8 GBq, a 57% clinical benefit, including stabilization and minor responses (SWOG criteria), was observed. Objective responses were described in 5%. The most relevant finding of the study was the observed overall survival, with a median value of about 37 months and a median PFS of about 29 months. These results compared well with the 12-month overall survival of a historical group treated with ^{111}In-pentetreotide. The median PFS in this group was 29 months. Characteristically, patients stable at baseline had a better overall survival than those who were progressive at baseline. The extent of disease at baseline was also a predictive factor for survival.[42]

The results of 2 phase I–II studies and a retrospective evaluation in 141 patients were published by the Milan group in 2004. Somatostatin receptor-positive tumors, mainly gastroenteropancreatic and bronchial NETs, were treated with a cumulative activity of 7.4 to 26.4 GBq of ^{90}Y-octreotide, divided into 2 to 16 cycles, administered 4 to 6 weeks apart. The objective response rate was 26%, including partial and complete responses (SWOG criteria). Disease stabilization was observed in 55% and disease progression in 18%. The mean duration of response ranged from 2 to 59 months (median 18). Most who responded had GEP-NETs. A significant observation was that assessment of the objective response according to the basal status indicated that individuals stable at baseline demonstrated a better outcome (partial and complete responses in 32%) than individuals with progressive disease (partial and complete responses in 24%). In this series, 11 patients with bronchial tumors were included. Ninety-one percent were in progression at enrollment and were treated with standard courses of PRRT, with cumulative activities ranging from 8 to 22.5 GBq. After completion of the treatment, 1 patient had a partial remission and 8 patients showed stabilization of disease (SWOG criteria). In an earlier escalation study published by the same group in patients with somatostatin-positive tumors (mainly in progression), 3 patients with bronchial NETs were included, with resulting stability and partial remission in 2 patients.[28,29]

A multicenter study published by Bushnell and colleagues[30] in 2010 evaluated the role of ^{90}Y-octreotide in 90 patients with symptomatic, metastatic "carcinoids" (small bowel NETs). The data indicated stabilization of tumor response (SWOG criteria) in 74% as well as a durable amelioration of symptoms related to the tumor mass and the hypersecretion of bioactive amines. This trial reported a PFS of 16 months and an overall survival of 27 months.

More recently, the Basel group published the results of an open-label phase II trial in 1109 patients treated with ^{90}Y-octreotide, divided into multiple cycles of 3.7 GBq/m^2 each. Objective morphologic responses (Response Evaluation Criteria In Solid Tumors [RECIST] criteria) were observed in 378 (34.1%), biochemical responses in 172 (15.5%), and symptomatic responses in 329 (29.7%). In this series, the NET groups were 265 small bowel, 84 bronchial, and 342 pancreatic tumors. The rates of objective response were 26.8%, 28.6%, and 47%, respectively. A longer survival was correlated with tumor and symptomatic response. The best predictor of survival, however, was the tumor uptake at baseline.[31] Protocols combining ^{177}Lu-peptides and ^{90}Y-peptides have been recently considered to take advantage of the different physical properties of both 2 radionuclides. In theory, the combination of the 2 radioisotopes would allow simultaneous treatment of both larger lesions (based on the higher energy and penetration range of the particles emitted by ^{90}Y) and small lesions (based on the lower energy and penetration range of ^{177}Lu). This strategy, however, must still be validated in clinical practice in larger series. Furthermore, the previously published studies include treatment schemes wherein ^{177}Lu and ^{90}Y were administered using empirically designed protocols rather than being based on individualized dosimetric analyses.[47,48] The results of PRRT performed in a

Danish cohort of 69 patients treated in Basel with different combinations of Y-peptides and/or Lu-peptides were recently published. Complete response was evident in 5 cases (7.4%), a partial remission in 11 cases (16.2%), and stability in 42 cases (61.8%). The median PFS was 29 months. Pancreatic NETs responded better than those with small bowel tumors. Six patients with bronchial NETs were included: one exhibited a partial remission and 3 were stable.[40] Experience has also been obtained from studies with ^{90}Y-DOTA-TATE. A group of 60 patients with histologically proven GEP-NETs were treated with 4.1 to 16.2 GBq per patient (mean 3.7 GBq per therapy) in 1 to 3 cycles. Six months after PRRT completion, a partial response was evident in 13 patients (23%), whereas the remaining had stable disease (77%). The median PFS was 17 months and the median overall survival was 22 months. Hematological toxicity WHO grades 3 and 4 were noted during therapy in 10%, which persisted in 5%. After 24 months of follow-up, renal toxicity grade 2 was seen in 7 (11.6%) and the authors emphasized the need for careful renal monitoring.[39] The novel radiopeptide DOTATATE labeled with [177]Lutetium, ^{177}Lu-DOTATATE, or ^{177}Lu-octreotate attained great popularity since its introduction in clinical trials in 2000, reflecting its higher affinity for somatostatin S2, its easier manageability, a lower dosimetric burden on the kidney, and the possibility of obtaining scintigraphic images and dosimetric studies at the same time, owing to the γ photon coemission of [177]Lu. It is currently therefore the most commonly used radiopeptide for PRRT. The initial clinical trials were undertaken at Rotterdam University. In a preliminary report, 35 patients with GEP-NETs were treated with 3.7, 5.6, or 7.4 GBq of ^{177}Lu-octreotate, up to a final cumulative dose of 22.2 to 29.6 GBq, with complete and partial responses in 38% (WHO criteria). No serious side effects were observed.[49] In a subsequent amplification of this series, 131 patients with somatostatin receptor–positive GEP-NETs were treated with cumulative activities of ^{177}Lu-octreotate ranging from 22.2 to 29.6 GBq. In the 125 evaluated patients (SWOG criteria), a complete remission was observed in 3 patients (2%), a partial remission in 32 patients (26%), minor responses in 24 patients (19%), and stable disease in 44 patients (35%). Twenty-two patients (18%) progressed. Better responses were more frequent in individuals with a high uptake on baseline ^{111}In-pentetreotide scintigraphy and those with limited liver involvement. Conversely, progression was significantly more frequent with a low performance score and extensive disease at enrollment. Median time to progression was greater than 36 months,

comparing favorably to chemotherapy.[44] In addition, ^{177}Lu-octreotate treatment of metastatic GEP-NETs was also associated with a significant improvement in the global health/QoL on various symptom scales, particularly fatigue, insomnia, pain, as well as role, emotional, and social functions. The effect was more frequent in individuals with tumor regression, but, surprisingly, it was also evident in those with progressive disease.[50] Of note was the observation that there was no significant decrease in QoL in patients who were asymptomatic before therapy.[51] Recently, an evaluation of an enlarged series of 504 patients treated with ^{177}Lu-octreotate, 310 of which were evaluated for efficacy, confirmed the occurrence of complete and partial remissions in 2% and 28%, with minor responses in 16% and stability in 35%, respectively (SWOG criteria). However, the most significant information derived from this study was the impact of PRRT on survival, with a median overall survival greater than 48 months and a median PFS of 33 months. A direct comparison with data obtained from similar patients (in the literature) showed a substantial 40-month to 72-month survival benefit for PRRT-treated individuals. Although these data are not derived from robust/rigorous prospective randomized phase III trials, this substantial survival difference in all probability reflects a real impact of PRRT as a therapeutic modality. These PRRT data compare favorably with other treatments, such as chemotherapy, from both the cost/benefit and the tolerability point of view.[33] A categorization of objective response once again indicated that pancreatic NETs tended to respond better than other GEP-NETs, although functioning tumors (eg, pancreatic gastrinomas) tended to relapse in a shorter interval (median time to progression 20 months vs >36 in the remaining GEP-NETs).[44]

A cohort of 51 patients with unresectable/metastatic NETs, mainly of GEP origin, was treated in a phase I–II study aimed at defining toxicity and efficacy of ^{177}Lu-octreotate. Patients were divided into 2 groups, receiving escalating activities, from 3.7 to 5.18 GBq and from 5.18 to 7.4 GBq, with cumulative activities up to 29 GBq, based on dosimetry. Partial and complete responses were observed in 15 patients (32.6%). The median time to progression was 36 months, with an overall survival of 68% at 36 months. Nonresponders and patients with extensive tumor involvement had a lower survival.[34] A recent prospective phase II study included a cohort of 52 patients with advanced well/moderately differentiated pancreatic NETs who were treated with ^{177}Lu-octreotate. According to the absence or presence of risk factors for renal toxicity, such as hypertension or diabetes, patients were divided into 2 groups and treated with different levels of activity, full dose (21–28 GBq) compared with a reduced dose (11–20 GBq), respectively. Both regimens resulted in antitumor activity. However, PFS was not reached at the time of the analysis in the cohort treated with the full-dose regimen, whereas it was 20 months in those treated with reduced doses, suggesting the former scheme should be recommended, whenever possible.[52] A phase II study was performed in individuals with "poor responding" tumors, including bronchial and gastric NECs. Patients were treated with standard 22.2-GBq to 29.6-GBq activities. Despite the limited numbers studied, the observed objective response (SWOG criteria) was comparable to GEP-NETs. The bronchopulmonary NETs results were 5 partial responses, 1 minor response, and 2 stabilizations in 9 patients. In the gastric tumor group, there was 1 complete response, 1 minor response, and 2 stabilizations (5 patients). In thymic tumors, the series was too small to draw any conclusions. The authors concluded that, contrary to previous findings, PRRT was as effective in bronchial and gastric NETs as in GEP-NETs.[53]

A recent study using a salvage protocol with ^{177}Lu-octreotate was published by the Rotterdam group. Patients in progression were enrolled after an initial response to PRRT with ^{177}Lu-octreotate, administered using standard cumulative activities (22.2–29.6 GBq). In this series, 32 patients with bronchial or GEP-NETs received 2 additional cycles of ^{177}Lu-octreotate, with a cumulative activity of 15 GBq. A new objective response occurred in 8 patients (2 partial and 6 minor responses), whereas stabilization was identified in another 8. Median time to progression was 17 months. Both response rate and duration over time appeared lower than during the primary treatment. Nevertheless, this "salvage therapy" was well tolerated by most patients and should be considered a valuable option

for this category of patient.[54] In more recent times, in keeping with recent tendencies in oncology, PRRT experiences have been focused toward combination therapies. In particular, combinations of the radiosensitizer chemotherapy agent, capecitibine, with ^{177}Lu-octreotate have been undertaken. An initial study in a small group (n = 7) with progressive GEP-NETs reported encouraging results.[55] Patients were treated with 4 cycles of standard activities of ^{177}Lu-octreotate followed by capecitabine (1650 mg/m^2) for 2 weeks. No severe toxicity, particularly hand-foot syndrome or hematological/renal-associated toxicity, was evident. Objective responses were observed. A recent phase II study of progressive NETs (n = 35) was reported.[56] Patients were treated with 4 cycles of 7.8 GBq of ^{177}Lu-octreotate followed by capecitabine, 1650 mg/m^2 (2 weeks). A 24% objective response with a 70% stable disease and 6% progression without adjunctive toxicity (RECIST criteria) was observed.

PRRT Safety Profile

After 18 years of experience, it is apparent that, from the safety perspective, PRRT with either ^{90}Y-peptides or ^{177}Lu-peptides is generally well-tolerated. Acute side effects are usually mild with some of them related to the co-administration of amino acids (including nausea, and rarely, emesis). Others are related to the radiopeptide, such as fatigue (common), or the exacerbation of an endocrine syndrome, which may rarely occur in the treatment of functional tumors. Chronic and permanent effects on target organs, particularly the kidneys and the bone marrow, are generally mild if the necessary precautions, such as fractionation and attention to specific risk factors, are undertaken (**Table 2**).[31,35,40,45,57] In this respect, it is apparent that, using appropriate dosimetry, it is possible to deliver elevated

Table 2
Long-term toxicity after PRRT with either ^{90}Y-octreotide or ^{177}Lu-octreotate in GEP-NETs

Ligand (Ref.)	Patient Number	Follow-Up (mo)	Renal Toxicity (Creatinine)	MDS	Leukemia
[90]Y-octreotide[57]	41	15	0	0	0
[90]Y-octreotide[45]	39	6	3% Grade 2	0	0
[90]Y-octreotide[28]	40	19	10% Grade 1	0	0
[90]Y-octreotide[42]	58	18	3% Grade 4	1	0
[90]Y-octreotide[40]	53	17	0	1	0
[90]Y-octreotide[31]	1109	23	9.2% Grade 3/4[a]	1	1
[177]Lu-octreotate[33]	504	19	0.4% Grade 4	3	0
[177]Lu-octreotate[34]	51	29	24% Grade 1	0	0

[a] Toxicity grade measured on glomerular filtration rate.

absorbed doses to the tumor, with relative sparing of healthy organs, such as the kidneys and the bone marrow (**Table 3**).

Although acute hematological toxicity is usually mild and transient, permanent and severe bone marrow toxicity may be a rare event after PRRT, as bone marrow–absorbed doses are usually below the threshold of toxicity.[58] Delayed renal toxicity that may occur if the dose threshold is exceeded is permanent. The kidneys, as a consequence of their marked radiosensitivity, represent the critical organs, especially for ^{90}Y-peptides administration. Renal irradiation derives from the reabsorption of the radiopeptides at the site of the proximal convoluted tubules, with a subsequent accumulation in the renal interstitium, where the radioactivity exerts its action. Studies with external radiotherapy indicate a threshold of tolerance in the range of 23 to 27 Gy.[59] The recently introduced BED concept appears more accurate in predicting toxicity and thus represents a more universal cipher to express radioactive dosage, irrespective of the modality of delivery. The use of this parameter indicates that the renal threshold for toxicity after PRRT is approximately 40 Gy.[60,61] A critical issue in ameliorating renal toxicity is provided by the strategy of co-infusing positively charged amino acids, such as lysine or arginine. These amino acids competitively inhibit radiopeptide reabsorption with a consequent 9% to 53% reduction of the renal radioactivity dosage.[62,63] Despite renal protection, a generally mild loss of renal function occurs, with a median decline in creatinine clearance of 7.3% per year for ^{90}Y-octreotide and a median 3.8% per year for ^{177}Lu-octreotate.[64] Nevertheless, instances of severe, end-stage, renal damage are currently extremely rare. Previous instances, for the most part, represent residual events that occurred during the early usage of ^{90}Y-peptide PRRT, when administration used very high activities in the absence of renal protection.[65]

In recent times, it has become apparent that a higher and more persistent decline in creatinine clearance with the subsequent development of renal toxicity is more likely to occur in individuals with pre-existent risk factors for delayed renal toxicity. These risk factors include long-standing and/or poorly controlled diabetes and hypertension. PRRT with ^{90}Y-peptides in particular seems more frequently associated with a reduction of renal function; presumably, this reflects the physical characteristics of the radioisotope. In a long-term evaluation of renal toxicity after PRRT in a group of 28 patients undergoing PRRT with dosimetric analysis, 23 of whom were treated with ^{90}Y-octreotide, a low, 28-Gy BED threshold was observed in patients with risk factors (mainly hypertension and diabetes), in comparison to 40 Gy in individuals without such risk factors.[66]

In a retrospective series of 1109 patients treated with ^{90}Y-octreotide, 103 subjects (9.2%) experienced grade 4 to 5 permanent renal toxicity.[31] Multivariate regression revealed that the initial kidney uptake was predictive for severe renal toxicity. However, it seems likely that this relatively high incidence of renal toxicity is related to the high administered activities per cycle (3.7 GBq/m^2 body surface, namely, activities of about 6.4 GBq per cycle in a standard man) and to the fact that individuals with pre-existing impairment of renal function were not excluded from PRRT. A further consideration is that routine infusion of protective amino acids was not used in the earlier component of the study.[65] From a hematological point of view, PRRT is generally well tolerated. Severe, WHO grade 3 or 4, toxicity occurs in less than 13% after ^{90}Y-octreotide and 10% after ^{177}Lu-octreotate. Nevertheless, sporadic cases of myelodysplastic

Table 3
Mean absorbed doses for ^{90}Y-octreotide and ^{177}Lu-octreotate

Organ	^{90}Y-octreotide Mean (Gy/GBq)	13-GBq Course (Gy)	^{177}Lu-octreotate Mean (Gy/GBq)	29-GBq Course (Gy)
Kidney[a]	1.1–5.1	15–66	0.3–1.7	9–48
Bone marrow	0.02–0.2	0.3–2.6	0.01–0.08	0.3–2.3
Tumor	1.4–42	18–542	0.6–56	17–1624

Data derived from published studies[58] (with examples of standard full courses of therapy, using either 13 GBq or 29 GBq). In general, absorbed doses to normal organs (eg, kidney or bone marrow) are variable on an individual basis. Specific tumor-absorbed doses depend on the level of radioactivity concentration in individual lesions and increase with radioactivity accumulation in the tumor. Tumor doses themselves are also highly variable based on factors intrinsic to the tumor, particularly the density of somatostatin receptors on the tumor cell membranes, the dimension of the lesions, and the distribution of radioactivity within the lesions.

[a] Renal doses are calculated based on the use of renal protection with amino acid solutions.

syndrome (MDS) or even overt acute leukemia have been reported.[14,38] Although predicted absorbed doses are lower than the conventional threshold for harm, both acute and permanent bone marrow toxicity is a cause for concern, particularly with repeated isotope administrations.[14,24,29,34] Dose-finding phase I studies indicate that the maximum cumulative administrable activity per cycle of ^{90}Y-octreotide, with renal protection, is 5.18 GBq.[28] An additional important observation derived from dosimetric studies is that hyperfractionation can lower the renal and bone marrow dose.[58,66] No dose finding studies have been conducted for ^{177}Lu-octreotate. Investigations using the dose-limiting toxicity method were abandoned, because literature data indicated that 7.4 GBq could be safely used as a maximum activity per cycle. Similarly, dosimetric studies indicated the advantage of hyperfractionation in lowering the renal and bone marrow dose.[34,44,58,66] In a phase I–II study treated with escalating activities of ^{177}Lu-octreotate up to 7.4 GBq/cycle in 51 patients, no major acute or delayed renal or hematological toxicity was observed and cumulative renal and bone marrow absorbed doses were within designated safety limits.[34] ^{177}Lu-octreotate demonstrated a higher tolerability compared with ^{90}Y-octreotide, largely due to the physical characteristics of the 2 radioisotopes.

An additional, although rare, consideration related to symptom exacerbation should be noted. A minority of individuals with functional lesions (eg, carcinoid, insulinoma, or Zollinger-Ellison syndrome) is susceptible. Paroxysmal amplification of symptoms is a consequence of massive radiation-induced cell lysis and subsequent release of bioactive amines or peptides into the bloodstream after PRRT. Such rare events can be rapidly managed by administration of cold somatostatin analogues, β-blockers, dextrose, or proton pump inhibitor agents dependent on the specific syndrome.[67,68]

FINAL CONSIDERATIONS

PRRT with either ^{90}Y-octreotide or ^{177}Lu-octreotate has been demonstrated to be efficient and relatively safe provided the known thresholds of absorbed and BED are carefully observed (**Fig. 7**). The renal and hematological toxicity profile is acceptable and can be further defined, if appropriate protective measures (such as amino acid protection and activity fractionation) are undertaken.

PRRT has also been demonstrated to induce a significant improvement in the QoL and diminution of symptoms related to the disease in most treated individuals. PRRT has a median PFS of more than 30 months, which represents a substantial improvement in comparison with many other therapeutic strategies used in NETs. In particular, individuals responsive to PRRT with tumor stabilization or reduction (~75% of the treated population) demonstrate a significant increase in survival (40–72 months from diagnosis). For these reasons, despite the absence of the results of randomized controlled trials, PRRT is considered one of the fundamentally effective therapeutic strategies in the management of NETs. As such, this modality of therapy (PRRT) has been included in the

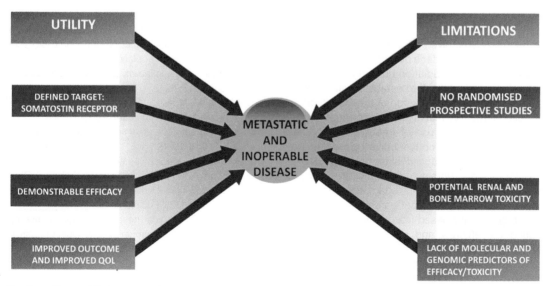

Fig. 7. Utility and limitations of PRRT in the treatment of NETs.

therapeutic algorithms proposed for NET disease management and has been accepted by the pertinent medical and scientific societies.[21,69–71] Despite such widespread acceptance and usage, there are several issues that require clarification in the near future. In particular, the precise timing of PRRT within the therapeutic algorithm of NETs requires delineation and reflects the relatively modest numbers of treated tumors, the relatively short follow-up, and the absence of randomized controlled trials. This critical limitation in defining the precise utility of PRRT will be addressed, at least in small bowel NETs, based on the outcome of a current ongoing multicenter study.

A further requirement in demarcation of the efficacy of PRRT is the need to more scientifically assess the parameters of response to the treatment. In particular, the specific molecular features of these tumors (indicators of radiation sensitivity), proliferative markers (Ki-67), and molecular indices defining response need delineation. Such information would further amplify the ability to assess efficacy beyond current parameters, such as evidence of disease extension, basal isotope uptake at receptor imaging, and morphologic assessment of the lesion type. Thus, pretreatment functional analysis of tumors using metabolomic parameters may convey information in regard to the likelihood of radiation sensitivity. Recent studies have noted that fluorodeoxyglucose (FDG) is a crucial parameter in predicting the duration of response to PRRT. Thus, individuals with positive FDG exhibit a significantly shorter PFS,[72] clear evidence that tumor glucose utilization represents a significant parameter in predicting therapeutic efficacy.

A further consideration is the assessment of the potential for renal and bone marrow toxicity. This area has not been rigorously investigated at a scientific level and remains a cause for concern among clinicians, given the potential for an effective therapy to engender a potentially critical series of adverse events. Radiation burden to tumor and normal organs is difficult to establish with acceptable accuracy, in the absence of the identification of individual factors that might redefine susceptibility. Alternatively, the use of treatment schedules with an excessively conservative approach, not considering the individual dosimetry and other biologic factors, may unreasonably limit the efficacy of treatment (see **Fig. 7**). In this regard, the delineation of molecular radiobiological parameters and individual, genetically based features inherent to predicting the efficacy and safety of radiopeptide therapy, would expedite the development of patient-specific and tumor-specific personalized therapy. The establishment of a profile of molecular determinants of both efficacy and toxicity would

facilitate the use of the most efficient tumor irradiation and, at the same time, define the most conservative safety profile with respect to normal organs.

REFERENCES

1. Modlin IM, Oberg K, Chung DC, et al. Gastroenteropancreatic neuroendocrine tumours. Lancet Oncol 2008;9:61–72.
2. Clark OH, Benson AB 3rd, Berlin JD, et al. NCCN Clinical Practice Guidelines in Oncology: neuroendocrine tumors. J Natl Compr Canc Netw 2009;7: 712–47.
3. Mallory GW, Fang S, Giannini C, et al. Brain carcinoid metastases: outcomes and prognostic factors. J Neurosurg 2013;118:889–95. http://dx.doi.org/10.3171/2013.1.JNS121556.
4. Frilling A, Modlin I, Kidd M, et al. Recommendations for management of patients with neuroendocrine liver metastases. Lancet Oncol 2014;15(1): e8–21.
5. Saxena A, Chua TC, Sarkar A, et al. Progression and survival results after radical hepatic metastasectomy of indolent advanced neuroendocrine neoplasms (NENs) supports an aggressive surgical approach. Surgery 2011;149:209–20.
6. Pape UF, Berndt U, Muller-Nordhorn J, et al. Prognostic factors of long-term outcome in gastroenteropancreatic neuroendocrine tumours. Endocr Relat Cancer 2008;15:1083–97.
7. McDermott EW, Guduric B, Brennan MF. Prognostic variables in patients with gastrointestinal carcinoid tumours. Br J Surg 1994;81:1007–9.
8. Rindi G, D'Adda T, Froio E, et al. Prognostic factors in gastrointestinal endocrine tumors. Endocr Pathol 2007;18:145–9.
9. Pavel M, Baudin E, Couvelard A, et al. ENETS Consensus Guidelines for the management of patients with liver and other distant metastases from neuroendocrine neoplasms of foregut, midgut, hindgut, and unknown primary. Neuroendocrinology 2012;95:157–76.
10. Modlin IM, Moss SF, Chung DC, et al. Priorities for improving the management of gastroenteropancreatic neuroendocrine tumors. J Natl Cancer Inst 2008;100:1282–9.
11. Weber HC. Medical treatment of neuroendocrine tumours. Curr Opin Endocrinol Diabetes Obes 2013;20:27–31. http://dx.doi.org/10.1097/MED.1090b1013e32835c32034f.
12. Doherty G. Surgical treatment of neuroendocrine tumors (including carcinoid). Curr Opin Endocrinol Diabetes Obes 2013;20:32–6. http://dx.doi.org/10.1097/MED.1090b1013e32835b32837efa.
13. Stevenson R, Libutti SK, Saif MW. Novel agents in gastroenteropancreatic neuroendocrine tumors.

JOP 2013;14:152–4. http://dx.doi.org/10.6092/1590-8577/1470.

14. Kwekkeboom DJ, Mueller-Brand J, Paganelli G, et al. Overview of results of peptide receptor radionuclide therapy with 3 radiolabeled somatostatin analogs. J Nucl Med 2005;46(Suppl 1):62S–6S.

15. Turner NC, Strauss SJ, Sarker D, et al. Chemotherapy with 5-fluorouracil, cisplatin and streptozocin for neuroendocrine tumours. Br J Cancer 2010; 102:1106–12.

16. Ramage JK, Ahmed A, Ardill J, et al. Guidelines for the management of gastroenteropancreatic neuroendocrine (including carcinoid) tumours (NETs). Gut 2012;61:6–32.

17. Reubi JC, Schär JC, Waser B, et al. Affinity profiles for human somatostatin receptor subtypes SST1-SST5 of somatostatin radiotracers selected for scintigraphic and radiotherapeutic use. Eur J Nucl Med 2000;27:273–82.

18. Hofland LJ, Lamberts SW. The pathophysiological consequences of somatostatin receptor internalization and resistance. Endocr Rev 2003;24:28–47.

19. Rinke A, Müller HH, Schade-Brittinger C, et al, PROMID Study Group. Placebo-controlled, double-blind, prospective, randomized study on the effect of octreotide LAR in the control of tumor growth in patients with metastatic neuroendocrine midgut tumors: a report from the PROMID Study Group. J Clin Oncol 2009;27:4656–63.

20. Caplin M, Ruszniewski P, Pavel M, et al. A randomized, double-blind, placebo-Controlled study of Lanreotide Antiproliferative Response in patients with gastroenteropancreatic NeuroEndocrine Tumors (CLARINET) - European Cancer Congress 2013 (ECCO-ESMO-ESTRO). Amsterdam, Netherlands, September 27 – October 01, 2013.

21. Zaknun JJ, Bodei L, Mueller-Brand J, et al. The joint IAEA, EANM, and SNMMI practical guidance on peptide receptor radionuclide therapy (PRRNT) in neuroendocrine tumours. Eur J Nucl Med Mol Imaging 2013;40:800–16.

22. Reubi J. Peptide receptor expression in GEP-NET. Virchows Arch 2007;451(Suppl 1):S47–50.

23. Krenning EP, Kooij PP, Bakker WH, et al. Radiotherapy with a radiolabeled somatostatin analogue, [111In-DTPA-D-Phe1]-octreotide. A case history. Ann N Y Acad Sci 1994;15:496–506.

24. Valkema R, De Jong M, Bakker WH, et al. Phase I study of peptide receptor radionuclide therapy with [In-DTPA]-octreotide: the Rotterdam experience. Semin Nucl Med 2002;32:110–22.

25. Heppeler A, Froidevaux S, Mäcke HR, et al. Radiometal-labelled macrocyclic chelator–derivatised somatostatin analogue with superb tumour-targeting properties and potential for receptor–mediated internal radiotherapy. Chem Eur 1999;7: 1974–81.

26. de Jong M, Bakker WH, Krenning EP, et al. Yttrium-90 and indium-111 labelling, receptor binding and biodistribution of [DOTA0,d-Phe1,Tyr3]octreotide, a promising somatostatin analogue for radionuclide therapy. Eur J Nucl Med 1997;24:368–71.

27. Otte A, Müller-Brand J, Dellas S, et al. Yttrium-90-labelled somatostatin-analogue for cancer treatment. Lancet 1998;7(351):417–8.

28. Bodei L, Cremonesi M, Zoboli S, et al. Receptor-mediated radionuclide therapy with 90Y-DOTATOC in association with amino acid infusion: a phase I study. Eur J Nucl Med Mol Imaging 2003;30: 207–16.

29. Bodei L, Cremonesi M, Grana C, et al. Receptor radionuclide therapy with 90Y-[DOTA]0-Tyr3-octreotide (90Y-DOTATOC) in neuroendocrine tumours. Eur J Nucl Med Mol Imaging 2004;31: 1038–46.

30. Bushnell DL Jr, O'Dorisio TM, O'Dorisio MS, et al. 90Y-edotreotide for metastatic carcinoid refractory to octreotide. J Clin Oncol 2010;28:1652–9.

31. Imhof A, Brunner P, Marincek N, et al. Response, survival, and long-term toxicity after therapy with the radiolabeled somatostatin analogue [90Y-DOTA]-TOC in metastasized neuroendocrine cancers. J Clin Oncol 2011;29:2416–23.

32. Kwekkeboom DJ, Bakker WH, Kooij PP, et al. [177Lu-DOTA0Tyr3]octreotate: comparison with [111In-DTPA0]octreotide in patients. Eur J Nucl Med 2001;28:1319–25.

33. Kwekkeboom DJ, de Herder WW, Kam BL, et al. Treatment with the radiolabeled somatostatin analog [177 Lu-DOTA 0,Tyr3]octreotate: toxicity, efficacy, and survival. J Clin Oncol 2008;26:2124–30.

34. Bodei L, Cremonesi M, Grana CM, et al. Peptide receptor radionuclide therapy with (1)(7)(7)Lu-DOTA-TATE: the IEO phase I-II study. Eur J Nucl Med Mol Imaging 2011;38:2125–35.

35. Bodei L, Ferone D, Grana CM, et al. Peptide receptor therapies in neuroendocrine tumors. J Endocrinol Invest 2009;32:360–9.

36. Mizutani G, Nakanishi Y, Watanabe N, et al. Expression of Somatostatin Receptor (SSTR) subtypes (SSTR-1, 2A, 3, 4 and 5) in neuroendocrine tumors using real-time RT-PCR method and immunohistochemistry. Acta Histochem Cytochem 2012;45: 167–76. http://dx.doi.org/10.1267/ahc.12006.

37. Dale R, Carabe-Fernandez A. The radiobiology of conventional radiotherapy and its application to radionuclide therapy. Cancer Biother Radiopharm 2005;20:47–51.

38. Kwekkeboom DJ, Kam BL, van Essen M, et al. Somatostatin-receptor-based imaging and therapy of gastroenteropancreatic neuroendocrine tumors. Endocr Relat Cancer 2010;17:R53–73.

39. Cwikla JB, Sankowski A, Seklecka N, et al. Efficacy of radionuclide treatment DOTATATE Y-90

in patients with progressive metastatic gastroen-teropancreatic neuroendocrine carcinomas (GEP-NETs): a phase II study. Ann Oncol 2010;21: 787–94.

40. Pfeifer AK, Gregersen T, Gronbaek H, et al. Peptide receptor radionuclide therapy with Y-DOTATOC and (177)Lu-DOTATOC in advanced neuroendocrine tumors: results from a Danish cohort treated in Switzerland. Neuroendocrinology 2011;93:189–96. http://dx.doi.org/10.1159/000324096.

41. Paganelli G, Zoboli S, Cremonesi M, et al. Receptor-mediated radiotherapy with 90Y-DOTA-D-Phe1-Tyr3-octeotide. Eur J Nucl Med 2001;28: 426–34.

42. Valkema R, Pauwels S, Kvols LK, et al. Survival and response after peptide receptor radionuclide therapy with [90Y-DOTA0,Tyr3]octreotide in patients with advanced gastroenteropancreatic neuroendocrine tumors. Semin Nucl Med 2006;36:147–56.

43. Yachida S, Vakiani E, White CM, et al. Small cell and large cell neuroendocrine carcinomas of the pancreas are genetically similar and distinct from well-differentiated pancreatic neuroendocrine tumors. Am J Surg Pathol 2012;36:173–84. http://dx.doi.org/10.1097/PAS.0b013e3182417d36.

44. Kwekkeboom DJ, Teunissen JJ, Bakker WH, et al. Radiolabeled somatostatin analog [177Lu-DOTA0,Tyr3]octreotate in patients with endocrine gastroenteropancreatic tumors. J Clin Oncol 2005;23:2754–62.

45. Waldherr C, Pless M, Maecke HR, et al. Tumor response and clinical benefit in neuroendocrine tumors after 7.4 GBq (90)Y-DOTATOC. J Nucl Med 2002;43:610–6.

46. De Jong M, Valkema R, Jamar F, et al. Somatostatin receptor-targeted radionuclide therapy of tumors: preclinical and clinical findings. Semin Nucl Med 2002;32:133–40.

47. de Jong M, Breeman WA, Valkema R, et al. Combination radionuclide therapy using 177Lu- and 90Y-labeled somatostatin analogs. J Nucl Med 2005; 46(Suppl 1):13S–7S.

48. Kunikowska J, Królicki L, Hubalewska-Dydejczyk A, et al. Clinical results of radionuclide therapy of neuroendocrine tumours with (90)Y-DOTATATE and tandem (90)Y/(177)Lu-DOTATATE: which is a better therapy option? Eur J Nucl Med Mol Imaging 2011;38:1788–97.

49. Kwekkeboom DJ, Bakker WH, Kam BL, et al. Treatment of patients with gastro-entero-pancreatic (GEP) tumours with the novel radiolabelled somatostatin analogue [177Lu-DOTA(0),Tyr3]octreotate. Eur J Nucl Med Mol Imaging 2003;30:417–22.

50. Teunissen JJ, Kwekkeboom DJ, Krenning EP. Quality of life in patients with gastroenteropancreatic tumors treated with [177Lu-DOTA0,Tyr3]octreotate. J Clin Oncol 2004;22:2724–9.

51. Khan S, Krenning EP, van Essen M, et al. Quality of life in 265 patients with gastroenteropancreatic or bronchial neuroendocrine tumors treated with [177Lu-DOTA0,Tyr3]octreotate. J Nucl Med 2011; 52:1361–8.

52. Sansovini M, Severi S, Ambrosetti A, et al. Treatment with the radiolabelled somatostatin analog Lu-DOTATATE for advanced pancreatic neuroendocrine tumors. Neuroendocrinology 2013;97: 347–54.

53. van Essen M, Krenning EP, Bakker WH, et al. Peptide receptor radionuclide therapy with 177Lu-octreotate in patients with foregut carcinoid tumours of bronchial, gastric and thymic origin. Eur J Nucl Med Mol Imaging 2007;34:1219–27.

54. van Essen M, Krenning EP, Kam BL, et al. Salvage therapy with (177)Lu-octreotate in patients with bronchial and gastroenteropancreatic neuroendocrine tumors. J Nucl Med 2010;51:383–90.

55. van Essen M, Krenning EP, Kam BL, et al. Report on short-term side effects of treatments with 177Lu-octreotate in combination with capecitabine in seven patients with gastroenteropancreatic neuroendocrine tumours. Eur J Nucl Med Mol Imaging 2008;35:743–8.

56. Claringbold PG, Brayshaw PA, Price RA, et al. Phase II study of radiopeptide 177Lu-octreotate and capecitabine therapy of progressive disseminated neuroendocrine tumours. Eur J Nucl Med Mol Imaging 2011;38:302–11.

57. Waldherr C, Pless M, Maecke HR, et al. The clinical value of [90Y-DOTA]-D-Phe1-Tyr3-octreotide (90Y-DOTATOC) in the treatment of neuroendocrine tumours: a clinical phase II study. Ann Oncol 2001; 120:941–5.

58. Cremonesi M, Botta F, Di Dia A, et al. Dosimetry for treatment with radiolabelled somatostatin analogues. A review. Q J Nucl Med Mol Imaging 2010;54:37–51.

59. Cassady JR. Clinical radiation nephropathy. Int J Radiat Oncol Biol Phys 1995;31:1249–56.

60. Daly R. Use of the linear-quadratic radiobiological model for quantifying kidney response in targeted radiotherapy. Cancer Biother Radiopharm 2004; 19:363–70.

61. Barone R, Borson-Chazot F, Valkema R, et al. Patient-specific dosimetry in predicting renal toxicity with (90)Y-DOTATOC: relevance of kidney volume and dose rate in finding a dose-effect relationship. J Nucl Med 2005;46(Suppl 1):99S–106S.

62. de Jong M, Krenning E. New advances in peptide receptor radionuclide therapy. J Nucl Med 2002; 43:617–20.

63. Bernard BF, Krenning EP, Breeman WA, et al. D-lysine reduction of indium-111 octreotide and yttrium-90 octreotide renal uptake. J Nucl Med 1997;38:1929–33.

64. Valkema R, Pauwels SA, Kvols LK, et al. Long-term follow-up of renal function after peptide receptor radiation therapy with (90)Y-DOTA(0),Tyr(3)-octreotide and (177)Lu-DOTA(0), Tyr(3)-octreotate. J Nucl Med 2005;46(Suppl 1):83S–91S.

65. Cybulla M, Weiner SM, Otte A. End-stage renal disease after treatment with 90Y-DOTATOC. Eur J Nucl Med 2001;28:1552–4.

66. Bodei L, Cremonesi M, Ferrari M, et al. Long-term evaluation of renal toxicity after peptide receptor radionuclide therapy with 90Y-DOTATOC and 177Lu-DOTATATE: the role of associated risk factors. Eur J Nucl Med Mol Imaging 2008;35: 1847–56.

67. Davì MV, Bodei L, Francia G, et al. Carcinoid crisis induced by receptor radionuclide therapy with 90Y-DOTATOC in a case of liver metastases from bronchial neuroendocrine tumor (atypical carcinoid). J Endocrinol Invest 2006;29:563–7.

68. de Keizer B, van Aken MO, Feelders RA, et al. Hormonal crises following receptor radionuclide therapy with the radiolabeled somatostatin analogue [177Lu-DOTA0,Tyr3]octreotate. Eur J Nucl Med Mol Imaging 2008;35:749–55.

69. Öberg K, Knigge U, Kwekkeboom D, et al, ESMO Guidelines Working Group. Neuroendocrine gastro-entero-pancreatic tumors: ESMO Clinical Practice Guidelines for diagnosis, treatment and follow-up. Ann Oncol 2012;23(Suppl 7):vii124–30.

70. Öberg K, Hellman P, Ferolla P, et al, ESMO Guidelines Working Group. Neuroendocrine bronchial and thymic tumors: ESMO Clinical Practice Guidelines for diagnosis, treatment and follow-up. Ann Oncol 2012;23(Suppl 7):vii120–3.

71. Kwekkeboom DJ, Krenning EP, Lebtahi R, et al. ENETS Consensus Guidelines for the Standards of Care in Neuroendocrine Tumors: peptide receptor radionuclide therapy with radiolabeled somatostatin analogs. Neuroendocrinology 2009;90:220–6.

72. Severi S, Nanni O, Bodei L, et al. Role of 18FDG PET/CT in patients treated with 177Lu-DOTATATE for advanced differentiated neuroendocrine tumours. Eur J Nucl Med Mol Imaging 2013;40: 881–8.

Medical Treatment of Advanced Thoracic Neuroendocrine Tumors

Piero Ferolla, MD, PhD

KEYWORDS

- Carcinoid • Neuroendocrine tumors • Target therapy • Biologic therapy

KEY POINTS

- The bronchial tree represents one of the most frequent sites of origin of neuroendocrine tumors (NET), with a prevalence that reaches 25% of all the NET.
- Furthermore, they are the subgroup of NET with a higher increase in incidence among all the NET in recent years, mainly because of the development of new diagnostic techniques in the last 3 decades.
- Thymic NET share with the bronchial NET the same histologic subdivision but are much more rare (<2%–3% of all the NET).
- Both of these tumors may be associated with multiple endocrine neoplasia type 1 syndrome.
- Thoracic NET (TNET) is a heterogeneous group of neoplasm, ranging from the more indolent behavior of the well-differentiated forms (typical and atypical carcinoids) to the highly aggressive behavior of the poorly differentiated forms (large cell neuroendocrine and small cell carcinoma).
- These 2 groups require a clinical approach totally different in terms of diagnosis and, above all, treatment.
- Chemotherapy and radiotherapy are the treatments of choice in poorly differentiated forms, whereas biological (mainly somatostatin analogues) and target therapy (mainly everolimus). Peptide Receptor Radionuclide Therapy (PRRT) and temozolomide have shown efficacy in small series or in the subgroup analysis of larger trials. The clinical response to these drugs does not significantly differ when compared with other well-differentiated NET, including gastro-entero-pancreatic-NET; however, no specific trials have been performed before this year.
- The first large, prospective, randomized trial (LUNA trial) entirely dedicated to TNET is ongoing at the time of this publication.

INTRODUCTION

The bronchial tree represents one of the most frequent sites of origin of neuroendocrine tumors (NET), with a prevalence that reaches 25% of all the NET.[1] Furthermore, they are the subgroup of NET with the higher increase in incidence among all the NET in recent years,[2] mainly because of the development of new diagnostic techniques in the last 3 decades. Thymic NET share with the bronchial NET the same histologic subdivision but are much more rare (<2%–3% of all the NET). Both of these tumors may be associated with multiple endocrine neoplasia type 1 syndrome.[3]

Thoracic NET (TNET) is a heterogeneous group of neoplasms, ranging from the more indolent behavior of the well-differentiated forms (typical

The author was in advisory board or speaker in symposia for Novartis, Ipsen, Lexicon, Italfarmaco.
Multidisciplinary Group for Diagnosis and Therapy of Neuroendocrine Tumors, ENETS Center of Excellence, Umbria Regional Cancer Network, Via E. Dal Pozzo, Perugia 06126, Italy
E-mail address: pferolla@alice.it

Thorac Surg Clin 24 (2014) 351–355
http://dx.doi.org/10.1016/j.thorsurg.2014.05.006
1547-4127/14/$ – see front matter © 2014 Elsevier Inc. All rights reserved.

and atypical carcinoids) to the highly aggressive behavior of the poorly differentiated forms (large cell neuroendocrine and small cell carcinoma).[4]

The clinical management of advanced TNET always requires a multidisciplinary approach. Every decision on the therapeutic strategy should be taken in the course of tumor boards that allow the evaluation of the different possibility of treatment including, whenever possible, the surgical treatment of local recurrences. A referral to third-level centers dedicated to these tumors is always recommended.

The main aims of the treatment are the control of the tumor growth and the control of the secretory pattern of the neuroendocrine tumor cells whenever endocrine syndromes are associated.

The clinicians approaching the cure of these tumors should always take in mind that, also after curative R0 surgery, only an accurate and protracted follow-up may assure that patients have been cured (also in typical carcinoid). The peak of recurrences is, in fact, located after more than 10 years from surgery in typical carcinoids and within the first 5 years in atypical carcinoids.[5–7] No evidence is available, at the moment, supporting the use of adjuvant treatment after radical surgery; however, in some subgroups with worse prognostic factors, such as atypical carcinoids N1 or N2, the design of clinical trials dedicated to assess the possible role of an adjuvant treatment with low-toxicity drugs, like as somatostatin analogues (SSA), is urgently needed.

CONTROL OF ASSOCIATED NEUROENDOCRINE HYPERSECRETIONS

TNET are associated with clinically evident endocrine hypersecretions in a percentage of cases inferior to the gastro-entero-pancreatic (GEP) counterpart (about 10%–15% vs 30%); however, if the subclinical secretions are also considered, the percentage increases up to 25% of the cases.[7] Long-acting SSA represent the drug of choice in the control of most of the associated hypersecretions, including carcinoid syndrome, which, in TNET, are more frequently atypical.[6,8,9] It should be remembered that atypical carcinoid syndrome, if not recognized, may be associated with an high mortality rate. Although reported only in small series, the percentage of response to these drugs in TNET seems similar to the GEP-NETs. H_1 and H_2 blockers, loperamide, and symptomatic therapies may be used in association with SSA with the intent to control some of the symptoms. In atypical carcinoid syndrome, the use of steroids may be required in association with SSA to control bronchostenosis and carcinoid crises; it should

always be remembered that the beta-2 agonist may exacerbate the symptoms, increasing the degranulation of secretory granules. Teloristat etipirate acts as an inhibitor of the enzyme tryptophan hydroxylase. This drug is actually under investigation in the course of phase II and III trials to increase the percentage of control of the carcinoid syndrome in patients not completely controlled by SSA.[10] Furthermore, it will be of interest to assess if an earlier reduction of the circulating levels of serotonin in patients affected by NET may be associated with a prevention of some complication of carcinoid syndrome and if the supposed reduction of the fibrotic phenomenons inducted by high serotonin levels may be associated with an antiproliferative effect.

Ectopic corticotropin hypersecretion and consequent cushing disease, growth hormone releasing hormone secretion and consequent ectopic acromegaly, and inappropriate antidiuretic hormone secretion may be less frequently associated with TNET. The treatment in these cases does not differ from the codified standard treatment. In order to reduce the amount of secreting cells, debulking strategies may be considered of some value. These strategies include partial surgical resections, hepatectomies, locoregional treatments (both radiofrequency and chemoembolizations), radioactive microsphere, and PRRT. The addition of alpha-interferon to SSA has been reported to be of some value in increasing their efficacy. All the listed procedures should be evaluated in terms of the risk-benefit ratio in the course of a multidisciplinary tumor board.

MEDICAL THERAPY FOR PRIMARY TUMOR IN PATIENTS NOT CANDIDATES FOR SURGERY, IN MULTICENTRIC FORMS, AND IN PATIENTS WITH ADVANCED METASTATIC DISEASE

The first multicentric randomized prospective trial entirely dedicated to TNET (LUNA trial, ClinicalTrials.gov Identifier: NCT01563354), started in the last months of 2013, is actually ongoing and will probably complete the accrual within 2014. No other prospective trial focused on bronchial NET have been published; therefore, the only available results come from small retrospective series and from the subgroup analysis of a few larger multicentric studies that allowed the inclusion of TNET.

Since all the neuroendocrine cells originate from the same neuroendocrine diffuse system and share most of the biologic features, it is reasonable to speculate that some of the results obtained in other neuroendocrine cell like as in the ileal carcinoid may be applicable also in bronchial carcinoid.

SSA AS ANTIPROLIFERATIVE AGENTS

As discussed in the previous paragraph, SSA have been used so far for the control of the NET-associated hypersecretions. The antiproliferative efficacy of these drugs and their use also in nonsecreting tumors have also been postulated starting from the last decade of the last century. However, the widely diffuse clinical use was supported mainly by the clinical experience and by the reports of small retrospective series.

Two large prospective phase III studies focused on small intestine NET have recently clearly demonstrated an impact in terms of progression-free survival (PFS) of the long-acting SSA octreotide (PROMID study)[11] and lanreotide (CLARINET study).[12] Based on these data and on the lack of any other larger studies with any type of drugs, SSA seem, at the moment, as the most reasonable first line in the treatment of inoperable well-differentiated TNET (including multicentric forms).

The proliferation indexes (mitotic count and ki67), the grade of uptake at indium In 111 pentetreotide (Octreoscan), and the rate of radiological progression may be evaluated case by case in a multidisciplinary tumor board to better define the need of additional therapies in the clinical management of advanced disease.

The role of SSA in the treatment of multicentric forms and precursor lesions, such as diffuse idiopathic pulmonary neuroendocrine cell hyperplasia (DIPNECH), seems reasonable but needs to be evaluated in specific studies. The same consideration should be reserved for their possible role in the adjuvant setting in high risk of recurrences, such as in atypical N1 or N2 carcinoid, for which a clinical trial is absolutely needed.

When progressive disease occurs in the course of therapy with SSA, no standard therapies are available. When available, a clinical trial should always be preferred. The first international randomized trial specifically dedicated to thoracic NEN, LUNA trial, will clarify the efficacy and safety of everolimus and pasireotide, whereas a multicentric Italian trial assessing the safety and efficacy of the association between lanreotide and temozolomide will start within the end of this year.

TARGET THERAPIES

Everolimus alone or in combination with SSA has shown activity in the subgroup analysis of a large multicentric trial (RADIANT II).[13] Forty-four patients with bronchial NET were treated in the study. The PFS in the arm treated with the study drugs was more than 8 months higher than in the placebo arm. However, an imbalance in the subdivision between the two arms of the study does not permit a correct statistical analysis[14]; this result should be considered at the moment an indication of a positive trend requiring further confirmation. A similar trend was reported in phase II studies than in the results of the everolimus expanded access program. In these studies, the impact on PFS of everolimus seems more relevant for carcinoid tumors when compared with pancreatic NET, which are, at the moment, the only NET with a recognized indication for this drug.

Prospective phase III trials are ongoing in other similar NET (ileal carcinoids) with PRRT and locoregional therapies. Despite the lack of large trials, the analysis of a small subgroup of metastatic TNET shows a rate of response similar to that obtained in GEP-NET.[15] A large phase III study (RADIANT IV) including also nonsecreting lung NET has completed the recruitment and is actually ongoing. It will explore the efficacy of everolimus as a single agent when compared with placebo in patients with progressive disease. The LUNA trial entirely dedicated to TNET will assess the efficacy and safety of everolimus as a single agent compared with the association with pasireotide or pasireotide alone in patients with progressive disease.

Many other target agents are theoretically active or seem promising in the preclinical models or in single patients or subgroups included in other small phase II trials, but these preliminary results need further investigations.

CHEMOTHERAPY

The use of monochemotherapy or polychemotherapy in well-differentiated TNET has been associated with poor results in the last decades. The results reported in literature come generally from small series, and the papers' methods include several biases. The criteria of inclusion infact often comprised patients with different grade of differentiation, no information regarding the progression of disease before the start of the therapy and inadequate criteria of evaluation of response to therapy. The percentage of G3-4 toxicity was generally relatively high. The cisplatin-etoposide scheme that constitutes the standard first line in poorly differentiated tumors should be reserved in well-differentiated tumors to patients who become rapidly progressive or when a rapid control of the associated endocrine syndrome is clinically needed (in association with the drugs reported in the previous paragraph).

Temozolomide alone or in association constitutes an exception, although the results are reported in small retrospective series.[16,17] The first prospective multicentric trial entirely dedicated to

TNEN will start these year. It will assess the efficacy and safety of temozolomide in association with lanreotide. The activity of the enzyme methylguanine orto methyltransferase seems crucial for the efficacy of this drug; however, the 3 methods of evaluation of this activity present different limitations, and not all the reports were concordant in the correlation to the response to the drugs. Based on these considerations, it is probably not ethical at the moment to select the patients by these methods; in a clinical trial, an a posteriori analysis or the advent of new methods will better clarify the clinical indication on the selection of candidates for this therapy.

SUMMARY

Based on the evidence coming from small retrospective trials, and on the subgroup analysis of trials including pulmonary NEN, everolimus and temozolomide seem to probably be the best choice in progressive metastatic disease when progression occurs after SSA and may represent the first line of treatment and the treatment of choice in secreting tumors. Temozolomide seems theoretically preferable when brain metastases are present and when concomitant radiotherapy is needed for bone metastases.[18] The toxicity profile of everolimus allows a long-term treatment, whereas the use of the alkylating agent temozolomide is better limited to a maximum of 24 months.

REFERENCES

1. Modlin IM, Lye KD, Kidd M. A 5-decade analysis of 13,715 carcinoid tumors. Cancer 2003;97(4):934–59.
2. Yao JC, Hassan M, Phan A, et al. One hundred years after "carcinoid": epidemiology of and prognostic factors for neuroendocrine tumors in 35,825 cases in the United States. J Clin Oncol 2008;26(18):3063–72.
3. Ferolla P, Falchetti A, Filosso P, et al. Thymic neuroendocrine carcinoma (carcinoid) in multiple endocrine neoplasia type 1 syndrome: the Italian series. J Clin Endocrinol Metab 2005;90(5):2603–9.
4. Travis W, Brambilla E, Muller-Hermelink H, et al. Tumours of the lung, pleura, thymus and heart. Lyon (France): IARC Press; 2004.
5. Daddi N, Ferolla P, Urbani M, et al. Surgical treatment of neuroendocrine tumors of the lung. Eur J Cardiothorac Surg 2004;26(4):813–7.
6. Öberg K, Hellman P, Ferolla P, et al, ESMO Guidelines Working Group. Neuroendocrine bronchial and thymic tumors: ESMO clinical practice guidelines for diagnosis, treatment and follow-up. Ann Oncol 2012;23(Suppl 7):vii120–3.
7. Ferolla P, Daddi N, Urbani M, et al, Regional Multidisciplinary Group for the Diagnosis and Treatment of Neuroendocrine Tumors, CRO, Umbria Region Cancer Network, Italy. Tumorlets, multicentric carcinoids, lymph-nodal metastases, and long-term behavior in bronchial carcinoids. J Thorac Oncol 2009;4(3):383–7.
8. Phan AT, Oberg K, Choi J, et al, North American Neuroendocrine Tumor Society (NANETS). NANETS consensus guideline for the diagnosis and management of neuroendocrine tumors: well-differentiated neuroendocrine tumors of the thorax (includes lung and thymus). Pancreas 2010;39(6):784–98.
9. Faggiano A, Ferolla P, Grimaldi F, et al. Natural history of gastro-entero-pancreatic and thoracic neuroendocrine tumors. Data from a large prospective and retrospective Italian epidemiological study: the NET management study. J Endocrinol Invest 2012;35(9):817–23.
10. O'Dorisio TM, Phan AT, Langdon RM, et al. Relief of bowel-related symptoms with telotristatetiprate in octreotide refractory carcinoid syndrome: preliminary results of a double-blind, placebo-controlled multicenter study. J Clin Oncol 2012;30(Suppl) [abstract: 4085].
11. Rinke A, Müller HH, Schade-Brittinger C, et al. Placebo-controlled, double-blind, prospective, randomized study on the effect of octreotide LAR in the control of tumor growth in patients with metastatic neuroendocrine midgut tumors: a report from the PROMID Study Group. J Clin Oncol 2009;27:4656–63.
12. Caplin M, Ruszniewski P, Pavel M, et al. A randomized, double-blind, placebo-controlled study of lanreotide antiproliferative response in patients with gastroentero pancreatic neuroendocrine tumors (CLARINET). Paper presented at The European Cancer Congress, Amsterdam, Netherlands, September 27–October 1, 2013.
13. Pavel ME, Hainsworth JD, Baudin E, et al. Everolimus plus octreotide long-acting repeatable for the treatment of advanced neuroendocrine tumours associated with carcinoid syndrome (RADIANT-2): a randomised, placebo-controlled, phase 3 study. Lancet 2011;378:2005–12.
14. Fazio N, Granberg D, Grossman A, et al. Everolimus plus octreotide long-acting repeatable in patients with advanced lung neuroendocrine tumors: analysis of the phase 3, randomized, placebo-controlled RADIANT-2 study. Chest 2013;143(4):955–62.
15. van Essen M, Krenning EP, Bakker WH, et al. Peptide receptor radionuclide therapy with 177Lu-octreotate in patients with foregut carcinoid tumours of bronchial, gastric and thymic origin. Eur J Nucl Med Mol Imaging 2007;34:1219–27.
16. Ekeblad S, Sundin A, Janson ET, et al. Temozolomide as monotherapy is effective in treatment of

advanced malignant neuroendocrine tumors. Clin Cancer Res 2007;13(10):2986–91.

17. Crona J, Fanola I, Lindholm DP, et al. Effect of temozolomide in patients with metastatic bronchial carcinoids. Neuroendocrinology 2013;98(2):151–5.

18. Pavel M, Grossman A, Arnold R, et al. ENETS consensus guidelines for the management of brain, cardiac and ovarian metastases from neuroendocrine tumors. Neuroendocrinology 2010;91:326–32 [Clin Cancer Res 2007;13(10):2986–91].

Index

Note: Page numbers of article titles are in **boldface** type.

Thorac Surg Clin 24 (2014) 357–360
http://dx.doi.org/10.1016/S1547-4127(14)00060-7
1547-4127/14/$ – see front matter © 2014 Elsevier Inc. All rights reserved.

Moving?

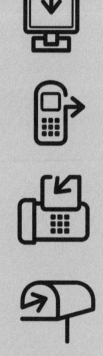